THE ENCYCLOPEDIA OF ESSENTIAL OILS

contains descriptions and usage information for

*Angelica	*Aniseed	*Basil	*Bay
*Benzoin	*Bergamot	*Birch	*Black Pepper
*Cajeput	*Camphor	*Cardamom	*Carrot Seed
*Cedar	*Chamomile	*Cinnamon	*Citronella
*Clary Sage	*Clove	*Coriander	*Cumin
*Cypress	*Eucalyptus	*Fennel	*Frankincense
*Garlic	*Geranium	*Ginger	*Grapefruit
*Hyssop	*Immortelle	*Jasmine	*Juniper
*Lavandin	*Lavender	*Lemon	*Lemongrass
*Lime	*Mandarin	*Marjoram	*Melissa
*Mimosa	*Myrrh	*Myrtle	*Neroli
*Niaouli	*Nutmeg	*Orange	*Palmarosa
*Parsley	*Patchouli	*Peppermint	*Petitgrain
*Pine	*Rockrose	*Rose	*Rosemary
*Rosewood	*Sage	*Sandalwood	*Tangerine
*Tarragon	*Tea Tree	*Thyme	*Tonka Bean
*Tuberose	*Valerian	*Vanilla	*Verbena
*Vetiver	*Violet	*Yarrow	*Ylang-ylang

Plus everything you need to know to use nature's oils to restore, revitalize, and rejuvenate!

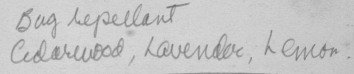

Bug Repellant
Cedarwood, Lavender, Lemon.

PRACTICAL
AROMATHERAPY

PRACTICAL AROMATHERAPY

Understanding and Using
Essential Oils to Heal
the Mind and Body

Robyn M. Feller

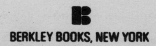

BERKLEY BOOKS, NEW YORK

PRACTICAL AROMATHERAPY

A Berkley Book / published by arrangement with
the author

PRINTING HISTORY
Berkley edition / April 1997

The Putnam Berkley World Wide Web site address is
http://www.berkley.com/berkley

ISBN: 0-425-15576-5

BERKLEY®
Berkley Books are published by The Berkley Publishing Group,
200 Madison Avenue, New York, New York 10016.
Berkley and the "B" design are trademarks
belonging to Berkley Publishing Corporation.

PRINTED IN THE UNITED STATES OF AMERICA

10 9 8 7 6 5 4 3 2 1

NOTICE

Medical research about the healing properties of different herbs is ongoing and subject to interpretation. Although every effort has been made to include the most up-to-date information in this book, there can be no guarantee that what we know about these herbs will not change with time. The reader should bear in mind that this book should not be used for self-diagnosis or self-treatment; he or she should consult appropriate medical professionals regarding all medical problems.

This book is dedicated to my love, Paul.

Acknowledgments

I would like to thank the many aromatherapy experts, friends, and family members who helped shape the direction of this book by taking the time to talk to me, E-mail me, and send me articles, including Dorene Peterson, Principal, Australasian College of Herbal Studies; John Kercher; Sheryll Ryan, District Director, National Association for Holistic Aromatherapy; Marcy Freeman of the Green Lotus Aromatherapy Company; Marcia Elston of Samara Botane in Seattle; Jim Dierking, Liberty Natural Products, Inc.; Douglas Wiggins; and all the members of my mailing list at aromatherapy@idma.com. I am most indebted to everyone who shared an anecdote, opinion, or a favorite aromatic blend. Special thanks, of course, to Hillary Cige and Jessica Faust at The Berkley Publishing Group—Hillary for thinking of me and Jessica for following through with her editorial insights.

Grateful acknowledgments to Elly Jesser-Yellin at Beyond the Crescent Moon in Great Neck, New York; Julia and David Rubel for their help early on in this project; Ivan Reich and Michael J. Feller for their advice; and to Elaine, Irv, Selma, and Sy for their loving support. And, of course, thanks to Paul for putting lavender on my pillow.

> Fragrant oil brings joy to the heart
> and a friend's support is as pleasant as perfume.
>
> Proverbs 27 v.9

PRACTICAL
AROMATHERAPY

Contents

Preface

As the interest in aromatherapy grows, there becomes a greater need to explain what this practice is—and what it isn't. It seems that every cosmetic company and health food store has a line of aromatherapy or aromatic products. How do you know what you want, what you need, and what you're getting?

In writing this book, I wanted to give the beginner to aromatherapy a basic reference to learning more about the tradition of this ancient practice and about the various essential oils that are used in aromatherapy. In the pages that follow, I have tried to give you a resource for understanding how to enjoy the many benefits of essential oils in a safe, effective way while ensuring that the products you use are of high quality.

Its feature characteristics are an easy-to-use Encyclopedia of Essential Oils, which is an alphabetical listing of essential oils used in aromatherapy, including a brief description of the plants they come from, how they are extracted, and what they can do for you; it also notes the other essential oils each mixes well with. Additionally, you will read about the best way to fully benefit from each particular oil. Also included are cautions so that the novice can use essential oils without harm.

Another feature is a section on choosing an essential oil. The modern (and recently omnipresent) world of aromatherapy makes for lots of confusion, especially for the uninformed. I have included a section on choosing what oil is right for you in specific situations. These wonderful oils with their many therapeutic properties will react with your system in different ways, depending on your physical condition and your mood. Provided for your convenience is an alphabetical listing of ailments, conditions, and moods and a brief description of which oils are best for each situation. Please note that my research is based on a great deal of existing literature as well as the findings of individual aromatherapy practitioners and users of this natural treatment.

One more note before we begin our journey: While aromatherapy is generally considered a safe treatment, there are some important cautions that you should keep in mind when experimenting with essential oils, since they are highly concentrated and volatile substances. Aromatherapy is a complementary medicine, not an alternative to modern medical care for serious diseases. It should, therefore, be used in conjunction with other treatments for serious illness.* If you are sensitive and have allergies, you may want to proceed with caution. If you are pregnant, heed the warnings in this book, but to really play it safe, get the advice of a professional aromatherapist before using any essential oil. People who suffer from such ailments as diabetes, epilepsy, asthma,

---

*Homeopathy can be contraindicated when using aromatherapy treatments. External treatments using camphor, mint, chamomile, black pepper, and eucalyptus should be avoided while being treated homeopathically.

and high or low blood pressure should also use care when using essential oils, as these substances can cause particular difficulties in those instances.

Remember, before there were synthetic drugs, there were herbal medicines. Essential oils are, indeed, powerful medicines. Treat them with the respect that Mother Nature deserves. Even too much of a good thing can be hazardous to your health. Use essential oils with care; essential oils have chemical compositions, just like other medicines. Aromatherapy is an applied science. We can isolate the properties of essential oils and therefore understand how and why they work to treat certain conditions. In fact, aromatherapy is not just about the odor of the plant and its oil, but the constituents that comprise each oil. Each oil has a unique aroma because of its individual blend of chemicals.

Although this book does list a great many physical ailments, it should be mentioned that Americans still look to aromatherapy as more of a mood enhancer and as a beauty treatment rather than a medical therapy. In Europe, especially in such countries as England and France, the medicinal benefits are more widely acknowledged. Given that, please be advised that the healing therapies in this book are based mostly on anecdotal information and traditional beliefs about the therapeutic properties of various plants and their essential oils. While there is more and more evidence that aromatherapy does have healing benefits, and many scientists and medical doctors do agree that aromas and essential oils have healing properties, the mainstream American medical community does not at this time acknowledge specific medical benefits. More research is being done all the time, however. Always seek qualified, professional assistance when using essential oils for any kind of medical treatment—that is, anything more than simple home use.

This book does not delve into the internal uses of essential oils. Although other books on the subject sometimes list aromatherapy treatments that can be taken orally, I have chosen not to include these practices here. This is a practice that arose among French aromatherapists, who are trained medical doctors, something that is not true of most American aromatherapy practitioners. It is generally accepted that without extensive training in the properties of essential oils and a deep understanding of human physiology, ingesting essential oils is risky business, at best.

I hope that, as you begin your introduction to the fascinating world of essential oils, you will find ways to derive pleasure and well-being from their powers. I truly believe that if you allow yourself to be open to the wonders of aromatherapy, you will experience great mental, physical, and emotional enrichment.

Smell is the sense of the imagination.

Jean Jacques Rousseau

Introduction

WHAT IS AROMATHERAPY?

WHY LEARN ABOUT AROMATHERAPY?

Cleopatra knew the power and allure of flower and plant oils. Madame Pompadour, Napoleon, and Josephine knew it, too. Now the modern world is embracing the ancient practice of aromatherapy with great enthusiasm. Aromatherapy, or the healing use of fragrant essential oils (the volatile oils extracted from plants), uses the specific properties of these essential oils to enhance one's mood and to treat a multitude of emotional and physical ailments ranging from anxiety and depression to dry skin and allergies.

Aroma is but one element of the treatment known as aromatherapy. We're all aware of the powerful connection the sense of smell has to our psyche. How we react to a particular smell depends a great deal on the mental association it evokes. Whether it's the whiff of the first crisp autumn day that brings you back to touch football games in the backyard or the tropical aroma of coconut that lands you on a poolside chaise lounge, you know that scent is a springboard to mood and memory. Helen Keller once wrote,

> Smell is a potent wizard that transports us across thousands of miles and all the years we have lived. The odors of fruits waft me to my southern home, to my childhood frolics in the peach orchard. Other odors, instantaneous and fleeting, cause my heart to dilate joyously or contract with remembered grief. Even as I think of smells, my nose is full of scents that start awake sweet memories of summers gone and ripening fields far away.*

Scent also evokes quick responses, so the aromatic component of aromatherapy actually can give you subtle yet immediate results. Who could walk through a beautiful garden with its medley of wonderful fragrances and not instantly feel better? Just smell the luxurious aroma of a fresh rose—you will almost definitely feel an instant sense of peace and relaxation. Smell is the fastest way to induce an emotional response. Need your sinuses cleared? Eucalyptus will do the trick. A quick sniff of lavender is usually all I need at bedtime to drift right off. (I recently misplaced my lavender vial and felt abandoned and agitated. Easy enough to remedy, however. Just another $7.50 and I was back in la-la land.)

The term *aromatherapy,* however, is somewhat misleading. This treatment goes beyond the sense of smell alone. In its truest sense, the healing practice of aromatherapy always involves pure essential oils and isn't limited to inhaling the scents as such, but it is a treatment that many people believe

---

*"Sense and Sensibility," *The Century Magazine*, LXXXV, February 1908, pp. 573–577.

has a chemical effect on the body and can be applied with massage and baths, as well as with skin and hair care. In Europe and other parts of the world, although not so much in the United States at this time, essential oils are taken orally for their healing properties. Aromatherapy is frequently used in conjunction with massage therapy, acupuncture, herbology, reflexology, chiropractic, and various other holistic treatments. If you've ever had a fragrant massage or relaxed in a lavender-scented bath, then you've already experienced some of the wonder of aromatherapy's magic.

RECENT INTEREST IN AROMATHERAPY

In America today, aromatherapy is gaining new momentum. Although it has been a popular treatment in Europe for quite some time, skeptical Americans have only recently acknowledged the tremendous healing benefits of natural aromatic cures. Research centers and mainstream medical facilities have begun to embrace the potential of these natural remedies, creating newfound enthusiasm and acceptance among the general population for this complement to traditional medicine, health care, and beauty regimens.

It seems that you can't pass a fragrance counter or flip through a beauty magazine today without being bombarded with new products claiming to be aromatics or containing essential oils. The healing properties of natural aromatic cures are big business these days, but they're not new business.

I recently attended a special seminar sponsored by The Aveda Institute in New York City, where Horst Rechelbacher, the founder of Aveda, spoke to an intimate crowd. He made a very interesting point about the perception of aromatherapy. He said someone had asked him if he considered himself to be New Age because of the type of business he runs. His reply was that no, he was "Old Age." His comment is very telling of the true nature of what aromatherapy is. It is, indeed, a practice that in its various forms has been around since the dawn of history.

THE HISTORY OF AROMATHERAPY

Aromatic plants and essential oils have been used for thousands of years for their healing and soothing powers, as well as for beauty, romantic seduction, and religious ceremonies. The word *perfume* comes from the Latin *per,* meaning *through* and *fumum,* meaning *smoke.* Perfumed incense, such as frankincense and myrrh, were often used in religious rituals and in the practice of magic in order to evoke the spiritual world. Incense, or the burning of gum resins from plants, is the origin of all perfumery.

When most people think about the aromatic uses of plants and flowers in perfumery, one woman comes to mind: Cleopatra. Cleopatra would fill her entryway with rose petals in order to seduce Mark Antony. In ancient times, it was routine to scatter rose petals at the feet of heroes. Rosewater was sprinkled on guests as they arrived at one's home. Cleopatra would drench not only her body in different fragrances, but even the sails of her ship were soaked in essential oils. Ancient Greeks and Romans used essential oils in their medical treatments. The Romans, especially, took to using essential oils for their beautifying and luxurious effects in bathing rituals. They would rub different oils onto different parts of their bodies both before and after bathing, as well as scenting their hair and clothes. Later in the historical timeline, we find Josephine covering her walls in sensual sandalwood to create a seductive mood for Napoleon.

Although the practice wasn't called aromatherapy until the early twentieth century, the use of essential oils actually dates back thousands of years. Archaeologists discovered a Mesopotamian distillation apparatus dating back over 5,000 years. It has been well established that Egyptians already used essential oils as early as 4000 B.C. and the Babylonians actually perfumed the mortar they used in building their temples. Clay tablets found around 1800 B.C. reveal an order for oils including cedar, myrrh, and cypress, essential oils that are still used therapeutically today.

Even in the Bible, Moses received the Lord's instructions (an early recipe?) on making a holy anointing oil. In Exodus 30: 22–25, the Lord tells Moses to take the following spices: 500 shekels of liquid myrrh, half as much fragrant cinnamon, 250 shekels of fragrant cane, 500 shekels of cassia, and a hint of olive oil. Given the therapeutic properties of these ingredients, this anointing oil would have been a powerful antiviral, antibiotic blend. Cinnamon is antiviral, antibiotic, and antifungal. Myrrh is antiseptic, too, as well as being a cicatrisant (promoting the formation of scar tissue). Unfortunately, however, the true ingredients are lost to us forever, since we cannot know for certain if the plants referred to in the Bible have the same botanical origins as the plants we know by those names today.

Ancient Egyptians often used aromatic plant essences to treat physical and mental health disorders. They used fragrant oils in perfumes, massage, baths, and religious ceremonies, too. They even used cedar oil in their embalming practices. Since essential oils contain powerful antiseptic properties, they would have been useful in slowing down the body's decomposition. In the East, ancient Chinese and

Ayurvedic (Ayurveda is the traditional medicine of India) doctors also acknowledged the therapeutic benefits of fragrant plant essences. Hippocrates advocated using herbs in baths, having said, "The best way to health is to have an aromatic bath and scented massage every day." As far back as 400 B.C. Hippocrates knew that burning various plants (incense), could offer protection from many contagions. Around that same time, Theophrastus, another Greek physician, wrote a treatise titled *Concerning Odors*, perhaps the first of its kind dealing with essential oils and what we now refer to as aromatherapy.

Steam-distillation was rediscovered in the late tenth century by Avicenna (980–1037 A.D.), an Arabian doctor, alchemist, and philosopher who is credited with the discovery of a method to distill essential oils from flowers, most notably from roses. This method also gave us rosewater, a less-expensive by-product of the distillation process of rose, which is still commonly used in health and beauty treatments. Avicenna is also an important figure in the history of aromatherapy in that his writings accurately described approximately eight hundred plants and their uses, as well as giving massage instructions that are so accurate that his techniques are used today. The knowledge about essential oils and fragrant waters was then brought to Europe from the East during the Crusades.

During the Middle Ages, essential oils and incense were burned in homes and in public areas in an attempt to conquer the Black Death and stop the plague's spread. Glove makers and perfumers of the time were said to have been protected from the plague by their use of essential oils in their work, especially since all essential oils are known to be antiseptic in nature.

By the seventeenth century, what Robert Tisserand calls

"the golden age of the English herbalists,"* knowledge of medicinal herbs was quite widespread, but had not yet been overshadowed by the science of chemistry and the spread of synthetic drugs, which would soon come onto the scene. By the eighteenth century, however, charlatans appeared, and the use of natural cures and herbal medicine declined. This, combined with the perceived need to lower costs, led to the beginning of essences being imitated with synthetic chemicals. Although still studied to some extent for their therapeutic properties through the nineteenth century, the use of pure essential oils and herbs for healing and in perfumes and cosmetics saw a great decline, and by the late 1800s, synthetic drugs became the norm to treat most maladies.

The modern concept and practice of aromatherapy actually begins with René-Maurice Gattefosse, a French chemist who, in the 1920s, coined the term *aromatherapie*. He was convinced that essential oils had powerful antiseptic properties—even more so than the known antiseptics being used at that time—as well as having other important healing abilities. Here begins the modern scientific research about essential oils and the most famous story about their amazing value. While conducting an experiment in distillation, Gattefosse burned his hand and needed to cool it with something. Serendipity struck; the only cool liquid around was a vat of pure lavender essential oil. He put his entire hand into the vat and found that the pain was gone almost instantly. Over the next several days, his burn healed with no blisters, scars, or infections. Gattefosse then began researching this incredible phenomenon and other possible medical uses of essential oils. His first book, entitled *Aromathérapie*, was

*Tisserand, p. 39.

published in 1928, followed by a number of scientific books and papers on essential oils.

With the outbreak of World War II, the study of essential oils was all but pushed aside. During the war, however, Jean Valnet, a French army doctor, used essential oils to treat soldiers' battle wounds when supplies of penicillin were low. Not much was researched or written on the subject until 1964 when Valnet wrote a book (also called *Aromathérapie*), which has shaped the basic ideology of our modern-day understanding of the use of essential oils as an effective therapy. Contemporary aromatherapy, as it was developed in France, is used to treat such ailments as insomnia, poor circulation, obesity, acne, sinusitis, depression, and stress.

Aromatherapy has recently been rediscovered in America and adapted by cosmetic and beauty companies, including The Body Shop, Origins, Estée Lauder, and Aveda, which refers to their products as "aromaology" products. It is generally more widely accepted in Europe as a complement to medical treatment, not just for beauty, hair, and skin care, but Americans are seeking alternatives to traditional health care options and are becoming more wary of putting synthetic chemicals into and onto their bodies for both health and beauty reasons, so aromatherapy continues to grow in popularity and acceptance.

When all is said and done, the appeal of aromatherapy is that you can help maintain good health and a sense of balance in your life through natural means, usually without risking serious side effects. In fact, most people experience little or no ill effects from the proper use of most essential oils. It is a treatment of guiltless pleasures, ranging from the inhalation of beautiful, fragrant aromas to calming, soothing, sensual massage.

Scientific research bears out that many plant essences can

help to induce a calm, relaxed state of mind. Aromatherapy, or using aromatic botanical essences as a natural remedy, can be as simple as dipping a cotton ball in the essences and inhaling, or dispersing the aroma into the air by means of an inexpensive store-bought diffuser. You can also blend these essences into a massage oil and apply it to the body. A mixture of lavender, geranium, and patchouli essential oils, for instance, relieves tension and anxiety; while chamomile and melissa act as antispasmodics and nerve sedatives. To treat stress, anxiety, tension, or mental fatigue, in fact, try any one or a combination of the following: basil, bergamot, camphor, cinnamon, clove, cypress, eucalyptus, geranium, ginger, hyssop, lavender, lemon, marjoram, neroli, nutmeg, peppermint, pine, rose, rosemary, or thyme. There are myriad options.

NATURE VS. CHEMICALS

To many, it seems strange to use these pure plant essences instead of synthetic chemicals for both healing and for perfume or beauty products. In the last century, we have become a truly petrochemical society. How odd that man-made substances are more readily accepted as good for us than nature's own. People in our culture often accept synthetic fragrances as better! Is it that we don't really understand nature? Prepackaged, synthetic perfumes are trying to imitate the real thing, so why not use the real thing? The first artificial aroma was born in 1838—bitter almond. By imitating nature, chemists actually tried to civilize nature and control it. But plant nature supports healing of human nature. Synthetics do not.

As we try to get back to nature, we must also proceed with caution. In the United States, the essential oil industry is not highly regulated, which is one of the reasons aromatherapy products do not usually make strong claims regarding medicinal uses. Also, since there is practically no regulation, it is difficult to know if what you're getting is the real thing. A product only needs about 1 percent essential oil to claim it contains pure essential oils. Some oils are of better quality than others. To ensure that you're getting what you pay for, especially until your nose is better trained, it is important to use reputable distributors, some of which are listed in the resources section of this book.

CHAPTER 1

What Are Essential Oils?

Essential oils are highly volatile, concentrated substances extracted from different parts of plants by such means as distillation and squeezing. These oils contain the pure essence of the plant from which they are taken and are often called the soul or the blood of a plant. For the plant, the essential oil's main functions are to keep the plant hydrated and also to protect it from predators. Essential oils contain many therapeutic properties, which might be antiseptic, antibacterial, or antifungal.

Essential oils are used in aromatherapy for the purpose of promoting physical, psychological, and mental healing through a variety of applications including inhalation, bath, and massage. There are hundreds of different essential oils. Approximately 70 to 120 are regularly used in aromatherapy treatments today.

Although essential oils are true oils, in general, they do not feel particularly oily and will not leave a greasy mark on a piece of paper the way a vegetable or mineral oil will. Like other oils, though, they do not mix with water, but they do blend very easily with vegetable oils, which is a common practice in aromatherapy for such applications as massage.

Essential oils are extremely concentrated and volatile, meaning they evaporate very quickly as they react with the air. When a bottle containing an essential oil is opened, some of the molecules escape as a gas, which then gets into your nose and you are able to smell the aroma. Some aroma categories follow.

Aroma Types

Citrus: of or pertaining to related trees or fruits
   Examples: orange, lemon, lime, grapefruit, and bergamot
   Aroma description: fresh, clean
Spicy: of or pertaining to spices
   Examples: cinnamon, clove
   Aroma description: heavy, sweet, deep
Floral: of or pertaining to flowers
   Example: rose, jasmine, geranium
   Aroma description: Light, semisweet, soft
Forest: of or pertaining to the bark of trees, the roots of plants, and woody plants
   Examples: sandalwood, rosewood
   Aroma description: woodsy, earthy, dry
Herbaceous: of, like, or consisting of herbs as distinguished from woody plants
   Examples: basil, sage, thyme, marjoram
   Aroma description: green and menthol

Feminine and Masculine

Sometimes aromas are described in terms of gender qualities. While there's no hard and fast rule, feminine aromas are marked by qualities that are generally attributed to women. Traditionally, floral aromas have been characterized as feminine. Masculine aromas are considered suitable for a man. Forest and spice aromas have traditionally been characterized as masculine. But let a man smell pure rose essential oil without seeing the label, and he might just go for it. In fact, in blindfold tests conducted by the Aveda Institute, American males loved the smell of rose when they weren't told the name of what they were smelling.

HOW ARE ESSENTIAL OILS EXTRACTED FROM PLANTS?

Aromatherapy is the art of using the power of fragrant essential oils to enhance your body, mind, and spirit. It draws on the healing powers of the plant world through the plant's essential oils, or the plant's soul, as the essential oils are sometimes called. The concentrated aromatic substance is located in tiny glands or scent globules found inside the various parts of the plants, including the flowers, roots, leaves, wood, buds, or fruit.

Parts of Plants	Examples of Essential Oils
Flowers	chamomile, rose, jasmine, ylang-ylang
Roots	vetiver, angelica
Fruits and seeds	coriander, caraway, cardamom, fennel, anise
Leaves	lemon balm, sage, thyme
Woody portion/bark	cedarwood, sandalwood, rosewood, cinnamon
Resin (used for incense)	benzoin, myrrh, sandalwood, frankincense
Fruit skin	orange, lemon, bergamot

When the oils are inhaled, they enter the body via the olfactory system (sense of smell). When they are diluted and applied externally, the essential oil molecules are believed to permeate the skin. In general, these concentrated essential oils have extremely small molecules, and therefore may be absorbed more easily into the skin than oils such as vegetable oil or mineral oil. The effects of using essential oils vary, but they are well known for their antiseptic properties and their ability to restore balance to the body, mind, and psyche.

The amount of essential oil that can be extracted from a particular plant is generally very small. The price of essential oils, in fact, is linked to the abundance (or lack of it) of the oil that can be readily extracted. It takes about two thousand pounds of rose petals to produce just one pound of rose essential oil, one of the most expensive oils used in aromatherapy treatments today. The method of extraction mainly depends on the type of plant. Nearly 80 percent of essential oils are extracted from the plant or flower by means of distillation. These include popular oils such as chamomile, lavender, and geranium. Others, such as the citrus oils, are commonly produced by a squeezing method. Try squeezing the rind of an orange or lemon; you will have extracted the tiniest amount of essential oil. Some of the more delicate floral oils are obtained through other extraction methods.

Regardless of the method, the oil that is extracted is going to be a volatile and highly concentrated substance that is made up of such elements as esters, aldehydes, ketones, acids, and alcohols. While modern science continues to try to fully imitate nature's oils, no one has yet achieved success. There is no substitute for the real thing.

The most common ways of extracting essential oils are listed on the pages that follow.

Methods of Extraction

Distillation

Many of us, when we think of stills, have images of the backwoods and moonshine, but stills go back in history as far as the second and third centuries A.D.

Distillation is the most common and economical method of extraction. The object is to produce an oil that is very close to the oil as it exists in the plant. During distillation only very tiny molecules evaporate, so they are the only ones that leave the plant. As a result, essential oils have very small molecular structures.

Distillation works in a fairly basic way. Plant matter is placed in the body of the still, which is filled with water. Steam then heats the plant material, and the essential oils are released, then evaporate. Together with the steam, the tiny molecules are carried along a pipe, which now contains the essential oil. As the molecules get farther from the heat source, a cooling process begins. The pipe passes through a container or vat of cold water and the essential oil condenses back into a liquid form. It will float on top of the water or, in some cases, will sink to the bottom. It is then removed for use in perfumery or aromatherapy.

In addition to the essential oil, another by-product of distillation is aromatic water (or flower water). This fragrant water is saved mainly when the essential oil is hard to come by, such as rose, neroli, and melissa. The process is similar to what was mentioned above, but to obtain a truly high-quality flower water, the same water is repeatedly piped through the system with each plant load.

Enfleurage

This is the traditional method used to extract flower essences, which tend to evaporate from the extreme heat of the distillation process. It is a time-consuming and therefore costly process, and so the resulting essences are very expensive, as is evidenced by the high price of jasmine and rose oils (absolutes) that have been extracted this way. At one time, pomades were produced by this process. Petals or leaves were placed on trays of animal fat for a number of days. Eventually the fat, which in effect was used as a solvent, was saturated with the plant extracts and would hold the floral fragrance.

Chemical Solvent Extraction

Absolutes, as well as resinoids, are produced by solvent extraction. Solvent extraction allows for the large-scale extraction of delicate fragrance materials at a moderate cost. The final products of this process, called absolutes, are very intense floral essences. This method is the preferred choice for such flowers as jasmine and violets, or with any flower that could not withstand the intense heat of distillation. It is important that almost all the chemicals are eliminated from the final product to maintain high quality. Traces of the solvents can, however, remain. Alcohol can sometimes be used as the solvent, which is generally the preferred method.

Expression or Cold-Press

This is the typical method used to extract the essential oils from plants in the citrus family. These oils are contained in the sacs under the surface of the rind. Better quality essential oils can be obtained from organic fruits, which are not sprayed with pesticides, since the toxic chemicals can make their way from the skin to the essential oil glands. Some large commercial fruit juice companies are now realizing the financial rewards of protecting the discarded fruit rinds of their product since perfumers and those who use essential oils for therapeutic reasons are more likely to want to use uncontaminated materials.

The shelf life of expressed oils is shorter than those that are distilled. It is therefore advisable to store them in a cool, dark place such as the refrigerator.

Carbon Dioxide (CO_2)

Essential oils produced by the carbon dioxide method are gaining in popularity within the aromatherapy field. In this method of extraction, carbon dioxide is liquefied under pressure to produce the oils, which in contrast to those extracted by distillation, have more complex aromas.

SIMPLE GUIDELINES FOR CHOOSING ESSENTIAL OILS: GETTING WHAT YOU PAY FOR

Aromatherapy and the use of aromatic substances in health and beauty products have become so widespread lately that it's hard for consumers to know if they're really buying pure, therapeutic substances. Quality is something that can be debated even among professionals, so your best defense is to educate yourself through experimentation and with expert advice. It is crucial that you use reputable sources (some suggestions are in the back of this book). Even among pure oils, though, quality can vary due to climate, country of origin, and collection and storage processes. Early on in your essential oil endeavors, you will need to trust your sources; as you become more familiar with the various oils, though, you can rely more on your own knowledge and instincts. With practice, you will begin to know what works for you. Most reputable suppliers are eager to know that they are getting good quality oils from their own suppliers. Many import directly from the country of origin. If you have doubts that what you're buying is pure or of good quality, it is your right and your duty as a consumer to go back to your source.

In fact, you can ask for proof of purity when buying essential oils. Consumers can obtain a certificate of analysis from an independent lab by calling on the manufacturer or distributor of any particular oil. Unfortunately, many essential oils that are tested are shown to be adulterated. By requesting this certificate, you can protect yourself from using oils that may contain some very irritating and unsavory bacterias and chemicals, such as ethanol, silicones, and benzine, to name a few.

Most reputable companies do quality control their inventory of oils and will be more than pleased to provide you with the information you request. The majority of American essential oil companies fall under the jurisdiction of the Code of Federal Regulations that deals with the cosmetics industry. Some of the things they monitor are sanitary manufacturing areas, compliance with labeling laws, and consumer safety. Just as you would expect to buy medication or cosmetics that have been tested for quality, you should expect no less from essential oil companies.

Also keep in mind that you can either choose to make your own blends or you can have them made for you through a variety of sources, including local aromatherapists, natural food stores, or mail-order suppliers, such as Aroma Vera or Aura Cacia. There are many other distributors nationwide and worldwide who can also supply you with good quality essential oils and carrier oils, as well as the application tools you need to do it yourself. For those not so inclined, however, many of these same companies create and market their own special blends for health and beauty purposes.

What About Cost?

Extracting pure essential oils is not easy business. Nature is not an unlimited resource, as much as we'd like it to be. It stands to reason that the more difficult an oil is to come by, the higher the cost will be to the consumer. It is for this very reason that you should approach the prices of essential oils with an educated eye—or nose. If you come across aromatic products made from different oils, yet the prices are all about the same, run the other way.

While some common oils, such as lavender, rosemary, or grapefruit, are relatively inexpensive, there are others that are so precious and rare that the prices are prohibitive to most. As an example, one ounce of grapefruit essential oil might go for about $10 retail. One ounce of French jasmine, on the other hand, might cost about $800. So the next time you see jasmine—just $9.95, you know you're not getting the real thing. Rose Alba essential oil from Bulgaria is another very costly oil. At over $1,000 an ounce, it is a prized possession, indeed. Cleopatra had good taste; she favored both rose and jasmine.

But take heart; there are many less expensive oils that can give you great pleasure and therapeutic benefits. For example, eucalyptus ranges from about $3 to $6 for a half ounce; lavender costs about $7 to $12 for a half ounce. If you crave something extra special, it is possible to buy very small quantities of the more extravagant oils. For just about $50, you can purchase a sixteenth-ounce bottle of jasmine. Often, a drop or two is all you need to receive the benefit of an oil, so a little bit can go a long way. Also, if you go to an aromatherapist, you can ask for a custom blend to be made especially for you. Often, they will charge you by the drop, so that touch of rose can be attained.

One last note about cost: it pays to comparison-shop for both price and quality. Price can depend on many factors, including the abundance of a particular oil at a particular time, import charges incurred by distributors, overhead—you name it. So do some research before you start buying so you don't get burned. Many distributors will be more than happy to send you a price list and product catalog at no charge. Some will even send free samples of essential oils.

Real vs. Synthetic

The consumer must not only be aware of price differentials among the pure essential oils but must also consider the real vs. synthetic question. How do you know that what you're getting is the real thing (an essential oil and not just a fragrance oil), and why should you care if it's real lavender essential oil or just lavender-fragranced smelly stuff?

It is certainly true that if something smells good to you, it can be beneficial, let's say, to bring about pleasure. An example would be all the mass-marketed perfumes out there. The key, though, is that those perfumes are trying to imitate nature. They are made up almost entirely of synthetic ingredients. The point of aromatherapy (key word *therapy*) is that the healing and mood-enhancing properties contained in these powerful and organic substances work *with* the chemistry of the human body in a natural process. Synthetics do not have the same benefits.

Go to any drugstore: the shampoo and body lotion shelves

are jam-packed with products claiming to be aromatherapy or aromatic blends made with pure botanical essences. While it might be true that there is a hint of essential oil in these products, you must be careful that you consider them for what they are—commercial products with, most likely, just a hint of pure essential oil. One of the challenges that exists for consumers in the field of aromatherapy, especially in the U.S., is that there aren't strong regulations about what can be called aromatherapy products. If it contains just the tiniest amount of essential oil, they can put it on the label. Aveda has an interesting approach to their products. They have decided to call their line of hair care and cosmetic products "aromaology" instead of "aromatherapy." They say straight out that they are a beauty product company; they are not trying to dose out medical assistance.

GENERAL GUIDELINES FOR USING ESSENTIAL OILS

The following suggestions are intended to help you obtain the best results from your essential oils.

- Use only pure essential oils. Do not substitute synthetic oils or aromas. (Quality differs among vendors, too, so do your homework.)
- Buy your essential oils and carrier oils from reliable sources (see Resources in back of book for suggestions).
- Because of the volatile nature of essential oils, never put oils near a flame or other very strong source of heat. The essential oil can actually burst into flames. Be especially careful when using a lightbulb ring. Also, do not add essential oils to a lit candle.

- Do not apply essential oils directly to your body. Always dilute essential oils in a carrier oil before applying them to your skin. Remember that essential oils are extremely volatile substances and are highly concentrated. Some are as much as one hundred times stronger than the fresh plant or dried herb from which they are extracted. Under most circumstances, only lavender can be applied directly to the skin (some say tea tree oil can, as well).

- When using an essential oil, uncap the bottle for only a few seconds. Since the oils are so volatile, they react quickly to the air and light. Always keep bottles tightly closed and protected from sunlight and heat when you are not using them. You can even store some oils, especially citrus, in the refrigerator.

- Use a dropper to place the oil into a clean, dark bottle or other container. It is important to keep the dropper and the rim of the container from touching your skin or other surfaces.

- Keep essential oils away from fine furniture. They can eat right through.

- Follow directions for aromatherapy blends carefully. Do not use more than the recommended drops of essential oil unless you are very experienced with the oils. (You can use fewer drops, however.) Remember, these oils are very strong substances. In general, less is more. You can always add more drops to a blend later on, but you can't take them out.

- Use glass containers for all blends consisting of essential oils only. Once diluted with carrier oils or lotions, you may have a bit more flexibility.

- If you must use a plastic container for an aromatherapy blend, be sure to add the carrier base oil/lotion or water to the container first and then add the essential oil or oils. Due to the highly concentrated nature of essential oils, they can damage a plastic container if not adequately diluted. Glass containers are always preferred.

- When using essential oils on infants or children, dilute the blend even more than is called for in recipes for adults. A general rule is to use half as much of the essential oil(s) in the ratio. Use caution when applying any essential oil to a child, especially babies. In fact, many experts advise not to treat babies up to the age of one with essential oils, but to use infusions of the herbs or plants instead.

- It is generally acceptable to shake a bottle of an essential oil blend to mix the ingredients. Be sure to keep the container well sealed. If you prefer a more gentle approach, either turn the bottle upside down a few times or roll the bottle between your hands for a few minutes.

- The nose knows. That old saying still holds true in aromatherapy. If an aroma is unpleasant to you, don't use it. Aromatherapy is really about bringing pleasure through the senses. If it smells terrible to you, all the books in the world telling you how lovely geranium is won't make you love it.

- Inhale essential oils for a short period only.

- If you have any reservations about any oil or blends you are using, *don't use them.* Trust your instincts. If you think you might have a sensitivity to a certain oil, you can do a patch test of the oil or the carrier oil blend by putting a drop behind your ear or in the crease of your elbow. Wait twenty-four to forty-eight hours to see if you have a reaction.

- If you experience any irritation, sensitivity, or unpleasant reaction, discontinue use of the oil in question.

- Never take essential oils internally, except under the direction of a health care professional who is trained in the medical use of aromatherapy. (This branch of natural medicine is practiced much more widely in Europe, especially France, than in the United States, where the medical benefits of ingesting essential oils in aromatherapy are still considered anecdotal.) This book does not give any recipes for the oral ingestion of essential oils.
- Store essential oils away from homeopathic remedies.

General Cautions

While topical and inhalation applications of essential oils are generally safe for most people if appropriate guidelines are followed, there are some instances when you should not use essential oils. People who suffer from certain medical conditions, including cancer, epilepsy, high blood pressure, low blood pressure, and those who are pregnant, must proceed with extreme caution when using aromatherapy. If you fall into one of these categories, always check with a health-care professional before using essential oils. Essential oils can counteract the benefits of certain other remedies, so if you are taking any homeopathic remedies, you should consult with a homeopathic physician.

Use aromatherapy treatments with caution under the following conditions:

- If you are under a medical doctor's care. (If you are being treated for a serious illness, get your doctor's permission before going for aromatherapy treatments.)
- During times of extreme fatigue or exhaustion. This might be a sign of more serious illness. See your doctor.

- If you have a fever or if your temperature is not normal.
- If you are suffering from a serious illness, including cancer, epilepsy, high or low blood pressure, diabetes, or if you are pregnant (consult a trained aromatherapist if any of these conditions are present).
- If treating specific problem areas, including recent scar tissue, infection, bruising, or inflammation, consult an aromatherapist. Also, proceed with caution if your skin is broken or if you are suffering from a recent break or bone fracture.

Allergic Reactions and Patch Tests

It is always wise to do a patch test before using any essential oil. Remember, these are powerful substances, so handle them with care. To do a patch test in order to test for skin sensitivity to particular oils, dot a couple of drops of your aromatherapy blend (only apply neat if using lavender or, possibly, tea tree) behind your ear or in the crease of your elbow. Wait at least twenty-four hours to determine whether your skin shows signs of itchiness, redness, or irritation. If it does, try a different blend of oils.

CAUTION: WHICH OILS NOT TO USE

The following essential oils are generally accepted as those that are unsafe for home use due to the strong possibility of side effects. They should only be used by trained aromatherapists, if at all. Some essential oils can be toxic, even in the smallest amounts.

Bitter almond	Orrisroot
Bitter birch	Pennyroyal*
Boldo Leaf	Rue

Calamus	Sage**
Yellow camphor	Sassafras
Cassia	Savine
Bitter fennel	Savory
Horseradish	Sourthernwood
Jaborandi leaf	Tansy
Lavender cotton	Thuja
Mugwort	Wintergreen
Mustard	Wormseed
Onion	Wormwood
Origanum	

The following oils must be used with caution under various conditions:

- Sage, aniseed, and hyssop are potentially toxic and should be used with extreme caution and only under the care of a trained aromatherapist.
- Fennel, hyssop, sage, and wormwood (which should be avoided completely) should not be used by those who suffer from epilepsy.
- Arnica, basil, birch, cedarwood, clary sage, cypress, fennel, jasmine, juniper, marjoram, myrrh, peppermint, rosemary, and thyme must be avoided during pregnancy. It is advisable to avoid lavender and rose essential oils during the first four months of pregnancy. It is generally accepted, though, that after that, these two oils may be used as 1–1½ percent dilutions. I recom-

---

*Pennyroyal is toxic and can cause miscarriages.

**There are mixed reports about whether or not to use sage essential oil. Generally, sage should only be used when under the care of a trained aromatherapist. Clary sage can often be substituted.

mend consulting a trained specialist before using any essential oils during pregnancy.

- Hyssop, rosemary, sage, and thyme should not be used by those who suffer from high blood pressure.
- Basil, lemon, lemongrass, melissa, peppermint, thyme, verbena, and possibly tea tree are considered skin irritants when used in the bath. They should always be substantially diluted in a carrier substance and also used sparingly—no more than three to four drops. For people who have sensitive or allergic skin, these oils should be avoided completely.
- Cinnamon leaf, fennel, fir needle, parsley seed, and thyme are considered skin irritants when used in baths or massage. They, too, should always be diluted in a carrier substance. No more than three or four drops in the bath and no more than a 2 percent dilution in a massage blend should be used. For people who have sensitive or allergic skin, these oils should be avoided completely.
- Angelica, bergamot, cumin, lemon, lime, orange, and verbena are known to cause photosensitization of the skin. Never use these oils on the skin before exposure to direct sunshine, tanning beds, or any other ultraviolet light. Serious burns can ensue.
- Marjoram, used to prevent spasms or convulsions, can be stupefying in high dosages.
- An overdose of saffron, a cerebral stimulant, can trigger convulsions, delirium, and even death.

For more specific information about possible dangers of essential oils, see individual listings in chapter 3.

CHAPTER 2

Using Aromatherapy

HOW AROMATHERAPY WORKS

Aromatherapy is the art and science of using essential oils extracted from botanical substances for the purpose of healing and balancing one's physical and emotional state. Essential oils contain chemically distinct properties that produce different therapeutic effects. The name aromatherapy is really a misnomer; it misleadingly implies that this practice is merely sensory in its application and effectiveness. While aroma always plays a role, the use of essential oils can take many forms, which includes not only inhalation, but massage, baths, and skin care.

The oils contain various minute chemical components, including ketones (found in chamomile, for example), esters (found in petitgrain and clary sage), oxides (found in eucalyptus), and aldehydes (found in bergamot). These components have properties that exhibit effects similar to those of synthetic drugs. For example, they could be antibacterial, antiviral, stimulants, or sedatives. When used properly, however, essential

oils are more compatible with the body's chemistry and healing abilities, and, therefore, produce few side effects.

Essential oils are approximately fifty to one hundred
times more potent then the dried source from which they are
extracted, so they must be used with care.

The Relationship between the Sense of Smell and the Rest of the Body

How does our sense of smell work so powerfully to affect
the way we feel? Scientifically, we know that aromas affect
our brain chemistry. When we breathe in fragrance molecules, they find a direct route through the nose to the brain
via nerve cells and transmitters. The molecules attach themselves to olfactory receptors that transmit impulses to the
various parts of the brain. Odor molecules influence the
brain's limbic system, which is sometimes called the old
brain or the olfactory brain.

The limbic system affects learning, emotions, memories,
and such physiological functions as appetite and sexuality.
Odor stimuli in the limbic system prompt the release of
neurotransmitters, including endorphins, which reduce
pain; encephaline, which promotes pleasant feelings; and
serotonin, which brings about a calm and relaxed state.
Specifically, the sense of smell affects the hypothalamus,
which controls the body's neurochemical and hormonal
regulation and is the part of the brain that communicates
with the sex glands; the frontal lobes, which control attention and memory; and the reticular system, which brings together the body and the mind.

Recent studies have shown that smelling certain aromas
does, in fact, have very definite effects. Rosemary, for instance, has been proven to decrease alpha brain activity, a

reaction that mimics the effect caused by a stimulating task. Aromas such as lavender, on the other hand, have been shown to increase alpha waves, which is similar to the effect of relaxation. In another study, conducted at the University of Cincinnati, subjects who inhaled the aromas of peppermint and lily of the valley while at work on a monotonous computer assignment made 25 percent fewer errors than those who inhaled unscented air. Maybe it's something inherent in those particular aromas, or perhaps it is simply that the scent made the people feel good, so they were able to work more effectively. In Japan, similar research was done using a lemon scent being piped into the air system in office buildings. The findings showed that the workers exposed to the lemon-scented air made over 50 percent fewer errors than those who sniffed only plain air.

In yet another study, conducted at Case Western University School of Dentistry at Cleveland by Ann Boyle, DMD, MA, associate professor of restorative dentistry, it was found that pleasant scents help reduce the anxiety of visiting the dentist. Patients undergoing root canal were divided into three groups. The first group was exposed to a floral scent, the second to a spicy scent, the third to no scent. The result concluded that the floral scent group reported significantly less anxiety than the other two groups. If you're prone to dental anxiety, then the key may be to wear a floral-based fragrance to your dental appointment.

Beating stress and burnout is probably the most widely accepted use of modern aromatherapy. Sedative fragrances, such as lavender, marjoram, and neroli (orange blossom) are among the oils in this category that are particularly valuable for relieving such stress-related symptoms as insomnia, anxiety, anger, irritability, and hypertension. These aromas prompt the production of seratonin. It has been documented that some antisocial behavior and hyperactivity in children is directly linked to a lack of seratonin. Euphoric scents, such as rose or clary sage, which stimulate the thalamus and the production of enkephlins, help to relieve emotional blockages. These aromas tend to help fight depression and moodiness. Stimulating scents, such as peppermint and rosemary, stimulate the production of adrenaline, which helps increase energy levels and fights mental and physical fatigue. Regulating scents, such as geranium, work on the body to balance hormones and to stabilize the psyche. These scents are particularly useful in battling mood swings, depression, and sometimes debilitating symptoms of PMS.

The uses of essential oils are numerous. Everything we have ever smelled, tasted, felt, touched, or heard, in fact, is stored in our brain through our life experiences. Because of those diverse human experiences, we all like different things. Aromatherapy, then, cannot be an exact science in terms of how aromas affect us emotionally. Although biologically we should respond a certain way to a particular aroma, we actually respond psychologically. Lavender, for instance, has wonderfully calming properties, and for most people, the scent will bring about relaxation; but if for someone the smell of lavender recalls some unpleasant memory, lavender will not have a calming effect. We are all products of our past. People like different things, so choose fragrances that elicit pleasurable feelings, regardless of what this or any other book might tell you.

When applied externally through massage, baths, or compresses, essential oils, due to their small molecular structure, are believed to be absorbed by the skin, the body's largest organ, and are able to enter the body's system through connective and lymphatic tissue, as well as the circulatory system. Creams, lotions, and other skin preparations are other applications for the use of plant essences. Regardless of the method of application, some oil will still be inhaled.

Here are some of the most common application techniques for essential oils and recommendations on how they can best be used.

USING DIFFERENT APPLICATION METHODS

Air Fresheners

Fragrance (Simmer) Bowls, Room Sprays/Other Air Fresheners

To diffuse the essential oil or oils of your choice into the air, add a few drops (up to eight or nine, depending on how large the room is) to a bowl of warm (not boiling) water. You can put the bowl on top of a radiator to further diffuse the fragrance into the room. A nice use for fragrance bowls is for setting a pretty table when company comes by. Add a couple of drops of a great-smelling essential oil, such as orange, rose, jasmine, or geranium (or one drop clove or cinnamon) to a sixteen-ounce bottle (500 ml) of springwater. Shake well and pour the fragrant water into decorative bowls and place on your dining table for a dinner party setting with a sensory punch.

Alternatively, you can add several drops to a clean spray bottle filled with water (usually four to six drops per eight ounces of water). Shake well before using and spritz into the air or on carpets, curtains, and furniture (except high-quality wood furniture). Or just sprinkle a couple of drops of the oil onto the carpet. You could also add several drops to a cotton ball and place it on a radiator. The heat will diffuse the aroma nicely.

Heat Diffusers

Ceramic diffusers come in different styles, but they all provide a gentle dispersion of aromatic essential oils into your environment. Ceramic diffusers all have a candle placed below a shallow bowl, which you fill with water. Then add a few drops of essential oil or a blend to the water. Light the candle. The heat of the candle allows the scent to be diffused into the air, creating a subtle, mood-enhancing environment. Be careful not to let the candle outlast the water or the bowl could crack.

Electric Diffusers

These devices continuously release minute particles of essential oils into the air at high pressure. The pumping action of air nebulizes the oils into small particulates. Some have metal reservoirs; others have glass. It is generally advised to follow specific manufacturers' instructions. Electric diffusers can be a good choice if you have small children or even small pets, as you do not have to worry about an open flame.

Lightbulb Ring

This is a ceramic or metal ring that sits on top of a lightbulb. Once the ring is positioned, place a couple of drops of your selected essential oil or blend in the ring. The heat of the lightbulb will vaporize the aroma into the room. *Caution:* This method can be potentially dangerous. Many users of this method report that the ring often slips off the bulb. Never add the essential oil while the ring is already positioned on the bulb. Also, if any essential oil drips onto the bulb or the fitting, you have a very real fire hazard.

Humidifiers/Vaporizers

Add up to eight or nine drops of an essential oil or synergistic blend to the water of a humidifier.

For the Body

Compresses (Hot and Cold)

Hot and cold compresses with essential oils can be used with great success to treat various pains and injuries. Hot compresses can be used with essential oils to reduce pain and swelling, especially when dealing with a chronic condition such as arthritis, back pain, and rheumatism. Hot compresses are also good for earaches, toothaches, and other dull aches. Cold compresses can be used with essential oils when there is inflammation to reduce pain and swelling, especially for acute pain and as a first-aid remedy for injuries and sprains.

Fill a bowl or basin with hot or cold water, depending on your situation. Add four or five drops of essential oil to the water. The essential oils will float on top. The compress should be placed into the water to absorb the floating oil. Gently squeeze out excess water and apply the compress to the affected area.

Hot or cold, it is best to use a cloth made from a natural fiber, such as cotton. Don't use too much water, just enough to soak into the compress. Try to keep the compress on the area for at least an hour.

Facial Oils

To create a nourishing facial oil, blend the desired essential oil(s) with a carrier (base) oil, usually sweet almond oil or grapeseed oil. The general rule is the mixture should be 99 percent carrier oil combined with 1 percent essential oil.

Massage Oil

Aromatherapy massage is one of the best ways to incorporate the healing powers of essential oils with the therapeutic benefits of touch. While the aroma and chemical properties of the oils serve to stimulate or relax the mind and body, the hands of the professional, friend, or lover massage away aches and pains and give the human body much-needed contact.

To create a wonderful massage oil, blend the desired essential oil(s) with a carrier (base) oil, usually a cold-pressed, nonprocessed vegetable oil such as sweet almond oil (see section on carrier oils). The general rule is the mixture should be 98 percent carrier oil combined with 2 percent essential oil (no more than 3 percent, or approximately 2 fluid ounces (50 ml) carrier oil with twenty drops of essential oil. This is for general-purpose blends. Blends for pregnant women or for those with sensitive skin should use only one percent essential oil.

Facial Compresses

Add three or four drops of essential oils to two pints of warm water that has been heated to boiling and then cooled. Stir gently. Take a small, clean washcloth and dip it into the water. Wring out the excess moisture and apply the compress to your face. Rose, geranium, sandalwood, lavender, and chamomile are among the essential oils that can be used.

Skin Toner

Add up to five drops of essential oils to four ounces of water. Use to refresh and tone skin.

Skin Lotion

Add approximately ten to fifteen drops of essential oil to four ounces of unscented, oil-based body lotion that does not contain mineral oil. *Caution:* Do not use cinnamon essential oil.

Perfume

Add ten to fifteen drops of your favorite oil or blend to one half ounce of jojoba oil or alcohol.

Hair Care

The following essential oils are especially beneficial for hair care: bergamot, carrot seed, cedarwood, cypress, chamomile, clary sage, frankincense, geranium, jasmine absolute, juniper, lavender, lemon, patchouli, rosemary, rosewood, sandalwood, and tea tree. Choose the essential oils you wish to use based on your hair type. For example, cypress, lavender, and bergamot are good for oily hair; lemon and Roman chamomile are perfect for normal light hair; rosewood, cedarwood, and lavender are particularly useful for normal dark hair. Dry hair benefits from geranium and lavender; dandruff sufferers might try eucalyptus or tea tree and rosemary. (Note: Erich Keller's *Aromatherapy Handbook: For Beauty, Hair and Skin Care* is a great resource for specific hair care recipes). The following homemade shampoo blend, hair rinse, and conditioner formulas are from Marcy Freeman of Green Lotus Aromatherapy Company.

Shampoo

To create your own shampoo base, try the following recipe: Add four ounces pure soap flakes, which you can purchase at a natural food store, to one quart of springwater. Heat the water to simmering, then add the soap flakes. After it is cool, pour into a clean jar or bottle for storage. Although it may start to clump up after some time, you can revive it by whipping it up by hand or with a blender. To make this recipe into a conditioning base shampoo, add one tablespoon of jojoba oil to the blend. You can use between ten and fifteen drops of any of the essential oils mentioned on the previous pages to create your custom shampoo blend.

If you don't want to go to the trouble of making your own base, unscented natural shampoo bases can be purchased from most sources that sell essential oils and aromatherapy products.

Hair Rinse

To make your own aromatic hair rinse, add two tablespoons of cider vinegar to one quart/liter of water. Add approximately ten to twenty drops of essential oil(s). Among those oils that are recommended for use in a hair rinse are clary sage, juniper, lavender, geranium, rosemary, patchouli, and lemon.

This formula is great to cleanse hair of buildup and residues. After shampooing your hair, apply this to wet hair and rinse with water. Note that vinegar tends to be drying, so only use it once or twice a week.

Hair Conditioner

To make your own hair conditioner base, try the following: Combine two ounces of liquid lecithin (a peculiar thick, orange substance that is available in health food stores), two ounces of almond oil, two teaspoons of jojoba oil, and one fourth ounce of cocoa butter. Using the water bath method (bano maria or bain marie), melt all the ingredients together until blended. Store in a jar when cool and add ten to twenty drops of your choice of essential oil(s) according to your needs.

A less complicated alternative is to simply dilute one teaspoon (5 ml) of your choice of store-bought conditioner, one teaspoon (5 ml) cider vinegar, and three or four drops of your choice of an essential oil or combination, such as patchouli, geranium, or lavender into two cups (500 ml) of warm water. Rinse through your hair after shampooing. Rinse clean for smooth, shiny hair.

Water-Based Body Applications

Baths

Bathing has been an important part of human existence since ancient times. Drainage systems were found in Egyptian and Indian excavations; since 4000 B.C., Egyptians used perfumed oils in their baths. Not just for religious and cleansing rituals, bathing was seen as a pleasurable and a healing activity. The great bathing halls of the Greco-Roman civilization contained a statue of Hygeia, the goddess of health. Hippocrates, in fact, advocated daily aromatic baths for their healing properties. The ancient Romans are the most famous bathers of history. They used scents for the pleasure of them, not just to mask unpleasant body odor, as most people believe. Taken to the extreme, as the Roman culture became more decadent, the public bathing rituals started to include sex. As we know today, when used in aromatherapy treatments, essential oils can, in fact, produce a sexual response as certain scents affect brain receptors in such a way as to activate the sexual glands.

Water and essential essences from plants are very complementary. Water, in fact, speeds up the activity of the oils, which is why it is so important to be sure that essential oils are well diluted in a bath, since certain oils can cause skin sensitivity and the water activates the oils.

Bath how-to: Get into a bathtub filled with warm water. After you've gotten used to the water for a few minutes and your skin is more receptive, add the essential oil(s) of your choice, usually between six to eight drops total. To ensure that the essential oil is properly blended into the bath for maximum benefit, swirl the water around with your hand. If you'd like, you can pour the essential oil into a small amount of shampoo, carrier oil, whole milk or cream, or even a bit of vodka (choose one that is high in alcohol content) in order to dilute the volatile oil, especially if you tend to have allergic reactions. Pouring the oil into an empty tub or under the running tap is not recommended since the oil is likely to evaporate before you even get into the tub.

Caution: Oils can make a tub slippery. Be very careful when getting in or out of the bathtub.

Sauna

Add one or two drops of your selected essential oil or blend to two cups of water. Using one cup of the aromatic water at a time, throw it on the hot rocks of the sauna, as usual. Eucalyptus, tea tree, or pine essential oils are generally recommended for the sauna because they readily enter the body through inhalation and leave the body via perspiration. These three oils are also known for their cleansing, detoxifying properties.

Shower

It's tough to use essential oils in the shower, since they are likely to evaporate too quickly for you to really get much benefit. One option, though, is to blend your own aromatic liquid soap for use in the shower. Using approximately four ounces liquid castile soap, add twenty to twenty-five drops of the essential oil or blend of your choice. Try using liquid soap on a loofah sponge.

Another option can be used before a shower. Add three or four drops of essential oil to a clean washcloth. Rub this all over your body and then take the shower as usual. Try equal parts rosemary, lemon, and eucalyptus or peppermint. After the shower, you can use a muscle relaxant oil blend or a toning oil blend.

Sitz Bath

Sometimes called a hip bath, this method can be used by adding approximately two to four drops of essential oils to a bathtub filled with just three or four inches of water (hip level). Also, there are specific sitz bath bowls made especially for this purpose. Be sure that the essential oils have been well dispersed before sitting down. Sitz baths are especially beneficial for treating hemorrhoids and thrush.

Footbath

Used by herbalists for hundreds of years, a footbath is a great alternative to a full-body bath. The soles of the feet absorb essential oils quite readily, so this is a quick way to experience the benefits. Add approximately two to six drops of essential oil to a bowl of warm water. Soak feet for twenty minutes.

Hand Bath

Add approximately two to four drops of essential oil to a bowl of warm water. Soak hands for a maximum of ten minutes.

Flower Water

Flower waters are produced as a by-product of the steam-distillation process during the extraction of essential oils from flower blossoms. The waters end up with beneficial properties from the flowers and often have rejuvenating effects on the skin. Rosewater is probably the best known flower water. In fact, rosewater is a nice alternative to the often cost-prohibitive essential oil of rose. Other popular flower waters include lavender and orange blossom.

The properties of flower waters are antiseptic, astringent, anti-inflammatory, and cooling. They are very soothing for the skin, especially for the face, when used in compresses and lotions.

Inhalation

Steam

The addition of aromatic essential oils can increase the long-held effectiveness of steam inhalation as a remedy for respiratory problems, including chest congestion, bronchial cough, bronchitis, laryngitis, and sinusitis. Inhale the vapors from approximately three drops of essential oil(s) that have been added to a bowl of steaming hot (not boiling) water. Eucalyptus and sage are among those particularly highly regarded for this purpose. Put a towel over your head and the bowl and breathe in through your nose. Facial steam baths can also be done following this method. *Caution:* Steam inhalation should not be used by anyone who suffers from asthma. Also, it is wise to keep your eyes closed. Do not use this method if you have any broken blood vessels.

Dry

Certain essential oils are beneficial if inhaled directly from the bottle. Alternatively, you can place one or two drops of an oil on a handkerchief or tissue and carry it with you and inhale the aroma as needed. To retain the fragrance when choosing this method, you can keep the tissue or handkerchief in a sealed plastic bag and open it when you want to inhale the scent.

Other

Insect Repellent Spray

Add five to ten drops of an appropriate essential oil, such as lemongrass, lavender, or citronella, to four ounces of water in a spray bottle.

Scented Pillow

For a peaceful night's sleep, place a couple of drops of lavender or marjoram essential oil onto your pillowcases before going to bed. Use eucalyptus oil when fighting a cold. *Caution:* Be sure that the oil is only used at the corners of the pillowcase so that it does not come in contact with your skin—or you might wake up with a skin irritation. While most essential oils evaporate easily and do not leave a stain, to be sure, use only those essential oils that are light-colored or clear.

Scented Linens

Using lavender, ylang-ylang, neroli, or another essential oil you choose, add two drops to a 500-ml bottle of spring water. Shake well. Pour the fragrant water into a plant sprayer and spray a fine mist over your bedclothes. If you prefer a stronger scent, add a few more drops of the oil to the water.

Scented Lingerie

Add ten drops of your favorite essential oil to a one-liter bottle of springwater. Shake well. Add a portion of the water mixture to the final rinse cycle of your washing machine or hand wash. Allow the lingerie to air dry, as a tumble dry can evaporate the fragrance.

Another alternative is to put a few drops of essential oil onto a cotton ball, store it in a small plastic bag, and tuck it away in your lingerie drawer. Many floral scents are good choices, such as ylang-ylang, geranium, jasmine, or rose.

Note: Some essential oils will stain clothing if applied directly onto the fabric.

Scented Ink

Choose your favorite oil. Add five drops of it to one teaspoon of ink. If using geranium, use two or three drops per one teaspoon of ink. If using myrtle, use ten drops essential oil to one teaspoon of ink.

Aromatic Jewelry

Aromatic jewelry is a popular way to use essential oils. Many essential oil suppliers are marketing pendants and earrings that hold essential oils. The body heat of the person wearing the jewelry allows the aroma to be diffused into the air, creating a great and creative way to keep your favorite scent with you wherever you go.

WHAT IS SYNERGY?

In aromatherapy, essential oils are often blended together to increase their effectiveness for treating particular conditions or creating certain moods. Synergy is the term used to describe the effect that is achieved when oils are combined to form a compound whose sum is greater than its parts. Synergy literally means working together, the phenomenon that occurs when two or more substances used together give a more effective result than any one of the substances used alone. The oils form a blend with a chemical makeup that can be substantially different from that of the individual elements.

The interactions of various oils have very specific effects on each other. Lavender, for instance, is known to increase the activity of other oils. Synergistic blends, therefore, can be very powerful substances and care should be taken with the amount of oils being used.

NOTES IN PERFUMERY

In perfumery, odors are classified into three categories, corresponding to notes on a musical scale. Piesse, a nineteenth-century Frenchman, developed a sophisticated ideology that each scent could be matched to a musical note. These notes, when properly combined, would form perfect harmony. Although the rules are more flexible today, perfumers still refer to scents in terms of the three classifications of notes: top, middle, and base.

Top or Head Notes

In perfumery, oils containing more of the smallest and therefore most volatile of the tiny molecules are known as top notes. Due to their volatility and therefore their quick evaporation rate, these odors by necessity have fresh, light qualities that are immediately noticeable in any blend—they're the first ones to reach our sense of smell. Examples of essential oils with top or head notes are tangerine, eucalyptus, lemon, bergamot, orange, lime, peppermint, verbena, and grapefruit.

Middle or Heart Notes

The middle notes, sometimes referred to as the heart of a fragrance, usually form the majority of a blend. In terms of volatility, heart notes are somewhere in between top notes and base notes. Middle or heart notes have soft, floral aromas that make their presence known after just one sniff. Examples of essential oils with middle or heart notes are clary sage, rose, ylang-ylang, tuberose, jasmine, geranium, hyssop, lavender, Roman chamomile, mimosa, myrtle, and neroli.

Base Notes

Those fragrances containing more of the heaviest and least volatile of the molecules are base notes. The scent is usually lingering, heavy, and rich, and it makes its way slowly and deliberately from the blend. Base note oils also act as fixatives for the lighter scents, so that they will not evaporate with such haste. Examples of essential oils with base notes are sandalwood, cedarwood, rosewood, pine, cinnamon, nutmeg, frankincense, angelica, juniper, patchouli, tonka bean, vanilla, and vetivert.

CARRIER (BASE) OILS

In almost all cases, undiluted essential oils in their pure form are much too concentrated to use directly on the skin. In many aromatherapy treatments, therefore, essential oils are blended into carrier or base oils. These oils dilute the volatile essential oil or oils so that you may experience the beneficial properties of the essential oils without irritating the skin. Especially for massage, where you need to cover a large area, carrier oils enable you to dilute the essential oils in proper dosages and rub them into the skin. In any blend, the base oil may be comprised of a single oil or a blend of oils (see the Professional Blend recipe on pages 52–53.

Carrier oils are generally vegetable, nut, or seed oils, many of which are familiar to us from cooking. The oils you want to use for aromatherapy, however, are not always what you find in the supermarket, as those oils may have been chemically processed. Oils that are labeled *extra-virgin, cold-pressed* are the favorite carriers to use. These oils are the first pressed oils from a particular crop and are the most beneficial to use since later extractions have usually undergone a heat or solvent process, which can destroy trace vitamins and minerals. Fixed vegetable oils are the most well known for aromatherapy purposes and essential oils dissolve extremely well in these carriers. Mineral oil (such as baby oil), on the other hand, is not a good choice since it protects the skin so much that it does not allow the essential oil to penetrate the skin. The most widely used in aromatherapy treatments is sweet almond oil, which is great for just about all skin types. Grapeseed oil, apricot kernel, peach kernel, and sunflower oil are other popular choices. These can all be used at full strength. There are other carrier oils that can be added as 10 percent dilutions, such as avocado oil or wheat germ oil, which are particularly good for people with dry or itchy skin (unless you're allergic to wheat, in which case wheat germ oil should be avoided). Most carrier oils used in aromatherapy have little or no aroma on their own, so they do not interfere with the benefits of the essential oils they are mixed with.

Essential oils, which are not really oily, but are volatile and evaporate quickly, are made up of very small molecules and can be easily absorbed into the system via hair follicles and sweat glands. In contrast, vegetable oils are made up of large molecules and will not be absorbed into the system as readily. Carrier oils, however, do have certain therapeutic properties of their own, and certain aromatherapy recipes call for specific oils for treating specific ailments.

Carrier oils also allow you to get more mileage out of precious essential oils. At full strength, a few drops of an essential oil will not go too far to cover the body, even if you could use it undiluted. But when added to a carrier oil, you can cover a much larger area and you will not have diminished the usefulness of the essential oil in the least. In fact, carrier oils may have therapeutic properties of their own that can enhance essential oils. Although massage is the main use for carrier oils, they can also be used for self-application of oils to particular spots on your body or to help essential oils to be dissolved in bathwater (see the section on Baths starting on page 29).

Remember that while essential oils are not greasy and most do not leave stains on sheets and clothes, vegetable oils do.

For the best results, it is recommended that you use carrier oils that are of high quality, just as you would choose for your essential oils. Here are the most common carrier oils that are used in aromatherapy treatment.

Sweet Almond Oil

This very pale yellow cold-pressed oil has been used since the days of ancient Rome where it was heralded for its ability to pamper and nourish the skin. Produced from the kernel, it contains vitamins and minerals and is extremely rich in protein. It is good for any skin type and is especially therapeutic for itchy, dry, or inflamed skin or for sufferers of eczema. It penetrates the skin particularly well, and it can be used full strength as a carrier oil. It keeps quite well, perhaps due to its high vitamin E content; it has a shelf life of approximately ten months. Sweet almond oil is one of the most used bases for aromatherapy blends for massage, bath, and skin care. It is great, even without essential oils, as a skin conditioner.

Grapeseed Oil

Grapeseed oil is practically colorless or sometimes has a pale, greenish hue. It is produced from the kernel. It contains vitamins and minerals and can be used on all skin types. It can be used full strength as a carrier oil, or is great when combined with sweet almond oil. It is lighter to the touch than many other base oils that are used in aromatherapy.

Avocado Oil

A good addition to an aromatherapy oil, the cold-pressed variety of avocado oil is cloudy, with a rich green color (in contrast to the pale yellow color of refined avocado oil). It is particularly beneficial for dry skin and wrinkles, and it contains vitamins and fatty acids. This oil keeps well as it is rich in antioxidant properties. Avocado oil can be used up to 25 percent in an aromatherapy mixture, no more than 10 percent in a facial oil. Some aromatherapists complain, however, of avocado oil's strong odor.

Apricot Kernel Oil

This pale yellow oil is produced from the kernel. It is chock-full of vitamins and minerals and is good for any skin type; it is especially therapeutic for sensitive, dry, inflamed, or mature skin. It can be used full strength as a carrier oil.

Hazelnut Oil

This yellow-colored oil is produced from the kernel. It contains vitamins, minerals, and protein. It is good for any skin type, especially dry, damaged skin, and possesses somewhat astringent properties. It can be used full strength as a carrier oil, and it is a particularly good choice as a base for sandalwood, rosewood, and ylang-ylang essential oils.

Jojoba Oil

This yellow-colored oil is produced from the bean. It is a very popular addition to base oils and should be used as a 10 percent dilution. That is, it should be combined with another carrier oil or alcohol, such as grain alcohol. It contains minerals, protein, and a waxy substance that is similar to collagen (jojoba oil is actually liquid wax). This highly penetrative oil is good for any skin type and is especially therapeutic for inflamed skin, eczema, psoriasis, acne, and in hair care treatments. Jojoba oil is usually the base oil in oil-based perfume blends as it does not go rancid as quickly as other oils. Jojoba can also be used to extend very expensive essential oils such as jasmine, rose, or sandalwood.

Wheat Germ Oil

This yellow/orange (some say red) oil is produced from the germ of the wheat kernel. It should be used as a 10 percent dilution. It has a thick, sticky texture, and it contains vitamins, minerals, and protein. It is an antioxidant oil that is especially high in vitamin E. It is beneficial for any skin type and is especially therapeutic for eczema, psoriasis, and prematurely aged skin. It has a shelf life of at least eight months and is often added to skin care products to help extend that product's life.

Caution: People who suffer from wheat allergies should avoid using wheat germ oil.

Coconut Oil

This oil, which is produced by pressing the coconut kernels, is often deodorized for use in aromatherapy treatments due to its strong scent. Coconut oil is best known for its use in tanning formulas and after-sun treatments and is reputed to filter the sun's rays. Coconut oil is often used in commercially prepared skin creams and lotions, as well, as it lends a smooth consistency to blends, but it can be irritating to sensitive skin and can cause a rash.

Calendula (Pot Marigold) Oil

This thick, yellowish oil is extracted from the flower of the plant. Calendula oil, known for its healing abilities for hundreds of years, is useful for the entire body. An excellent choice for basic skin care, it is especially beneficial for dry, chapped, and scaly skin. It is also used to treat varicose veins, bruises, and the chapped nipples of nursing mothers.

Evening Primrose

Evening primrose, a pale yellow oil, is a very good choice for face and body massage blends. It is rich in GLA (gamma linolenic acid), vitamins, and minerals, and it is especially healing for dry, dull skin and for skin with eczema or psoriasis. As a base oil, evening primrose should be used as a 10 percent dilution.

Sesame Oil

Sesame oil is a light, odorless, and inexpensive oil. It is especially useful as a base for massage oils containing essential oils with strong aromas. Sesame oil can be used on all skin types. Some claim that sesame oil is beneficial in treating arthritis.

Carrot Oil

Carrot oil is actually an essential oil, but it is frequently used in carrier oils. It is orange colored and contains vitamins, minerals, and beta-carotene. It can be used for treating prematurely aging, itchy, dry skin; eczema; and psoriasis; and it reduces scarring. It is also considered rejuvenating. Carrot oil should never be used undiluted on the skin. Use as a 10 percent dilution in a carrier oil.

Olive Oil

This well-known, strong-smelling, green-colored oil contains vitamins, minerals, and protein. It can be used in treatments for rheumatic conditions, hair care, and in cosmetics. It is excellent for its disinfecting properties and as a base for mixtures designed to care for infected skin. It is a very soothing oil that should be used as a 10 percent dilution.

Safflower Oil

This pale yellow oil contains vitamins, minerals, and protein. It is good for any skin type and can be used full strength as a carrier oil.

Corn Oil

This pale yellow oil contains vitamins, minerals, and protein. It is good for any skin type and can be used full strength as a carrier oil, although since this oil is almost always produced by hot extraction, it is not on the preferred list of most aromatherapy recipes.

Vitamin E Oil

Vitamin E oil is a very thick oil that is used in combination with other carrier oils. It is an antioxidant that can be used to extend the shelf life of other base oils and aromatherapy blends. It can prevent scarring and may fade existing scars if used regularly.

Soy Oil

Soy oil is a light oil with a mild aroma. It is absorbed quickly into the skin and can be used on all skin types. It does not aggravate acne or oily skin.

Sunflower Oil

Sunflower oil is high in vitamin E and is easily absorbed into the skin. It can be used on all skin types.

Borage Seed Oil

This pale yellow oil is derived from the seeds. It contains GLA (gamma linolenic acid), vitamins, and minerals. Borage seed oil should be used as a 10 percent dilution in a base oil. It can be used for eczema and psoriasis, as well as prematurely aged skin. It can also be beneficial for premenstrual tension and menopausal problems, multiple sclerosis, and heart disease.

Other Carriers

In addition to the base oils mentioned here, essential oils can also be added to store-bought body products such as shampoos, conditioners and rinses, body and hand lotions, and even powders. For skin care, some recipes call for such natural ingredients as aloe vera gel, honey, clay, vinegar, or milk. For the home, dishwashing soaps and cleaning solutions can serve as carriers for essential oils. Add essential oils to springwater to make room sprays or fragrance bowls, to alcohol to make perfumes, and to sea salt for fragrant bath salts.

When first experimenting, use a very small amount of essential oil (one or two drops), until you know what works for you. Save the expensive essential oils for use on your body; a less expensive version of lemon or frankincense is just fine if you're using it to clean your floors.

MEASUREMENTS AND DILUTIONS

In most cases, you should use no more than two to five drops of essential oil per teaspoon of base vegetable oil (1 teaspoon = 5 ml), which is usually a sufficient amount to massage an average person. Use one drop of essential oil to a teaspoon of base oil for use on the face. Here are some guidelines to help measure your blend of essential oils and carrier oils.

Essential Oil to Carrier Oil

1 drop	less than 1 tsp. (approx. ⅛ tsp.)
2–5 drops	1 tsp.
4–10 drops	2 tsp.
6–15 drops	3 tsp. (1 tbsp.)
8–20 drops	4 tsp.
10–25 drops	5 tsp.
12–30 drops	6 tsp. (2 tbsp.)

Measurement *Conversion Table*		*Essential Oil* *Conversion Table*
1 tsp.	5 ml	20 drops essential oil = approx. ⅛ tsp. essential oil
2 tsp.	10 ml	40 drops essential oil = approx. ⅖ tsp. essential oil
1 tbs.	15 ml	60 drops essential oil = approx. ⅜ tsp. essential oil
4 tsp.	20 ml	
5 tsp.	25 ml	
2 tbs.	30 ml	
7 tsp.	35 ml	
8 tsp.	40 ml	
3 tbs.	45 ml	
10 tsp.	50 ml	

More Equivalents

½ fl. oz. = approx. 15 ml
1 fl. oz. = approx. 30 ml
16.9 fl. oz. = approx. 500 ml

1 percent solution = 5 drops essential oil in 20 ml (4 tsp.) carrier or base oil or 2 oz. carrier oil with 20 drops essential oil/4 oz. carrier oil with 40 drops essential oil.

1 gram = 1 ml (approx.) = 20 drops essential oil (approx.) = 0.0353 oz.

Note: The size of a drop can vary from oil to oil and from dropper to dropper. It is very difficult to get a precise amount when using this method of calculation.

Understanding Dilutions

If a recipe calls for a 1 percent solution, that means that the essential oil is approximately 1 percent of the total liquid amount of the blend (i.e., 5 drops essential oil to 4 tsp. (20 ml) carrier or base oil.

The most commonly used dilutions are from 1 to 3 percent. Three percent is common for body and massage oils and healing oil dilutions, 1 to 2 percent is usual for skin care oils, and 1 percent is generally recommended for facial oils, for people with sensitive skin, and for children. For aromatherapy baths, six to fifteen drops of essential oil is the general recommendation, although some aromatherapy books call for stronger blends at the user's discretion.

THE BASICS FOR BEGINNERS

My first aromatherapy kit contained a small ceramic diffuser, half a dozen candles, and three small amber vials of essential oil—all for an initial investment of about $20. The accompanying literature said the lavender would help me sleep, the eucalyptus would clear my sinuses (and clear up a pimple overnight), and the rosemary would help with concentration, even provide relief from the worst malady, writer's block. Well, I'm well-rested, my nasal passages are clear as a bell, and this book is published.

When first starting to educate yourself about the many aspects of aromatherapy, you can begin with your local health food store. Many now carry some essential oils. Also, small stores specializing in aromatherapy and natural perfumery can be found in many areas, and herb stores, old-fashioned drugstores, fancy pharmacies, or mail-order suppliers can start you out. It's a good idea to read whatever you can on the subject and ask questions of knowledgeable store owners, distributors, and practicing aromatherapists. The aromatherapy beginner might want to consult a practicing aromatherapist for assistance in choosing oils, creating blends, and for general information about essential oils. If you do decide to go this route, be sure to check the therapist's certification; make sure he or she has taken an examination in the practice of aromatherapy. Also, check that the practitioner is a member of a professional organization, and finally, during your consultation, you should feel that the therapist is not just treating your symptoms but is seriously trying to uncover the source of your ailments.

Another great place to learn from the experts is on the Internet. There are literally hundreds of Web pages designed to provide aromatherapy information, as well as mailing lists and newsgroups where you can ask questions (even as a newbie) and receive the most up-to-date research and expert opinions.

Once you decide to get your feet wet, you will almost surely be hooked. Start slowly. Just purchase a few oils in small quantities. This will allow you to decide which oils you like and which work best for you, and it will also save you from waste. If stored and cared for properly, most essential oils can last many years, but light and air can do harm, so it's best to keep your quantities to a minimum. Most oils remain fully potent up to a year; after that they begin to lose their effectiveness. To maximize an oil's shelf life, it's best to fill the bottle to the top so that no air can get in and oxidize the oil. Also, avoid extreme temperatures (not below freezing, not above 95 degrees F). Citrus oils are among the most sensitive, so experts advise that they be refrigerated. Some essential oils actually improve with age, such as jasmine, patchouli, rose, sandalwood, and rosewood. To maximize the life of these oils, you can store them in the cellar.

Although there are about 700 different essential oils, between approximately 70 and 120 are commonly used for the majority of aromatherapy treatments. The following 16 essential oils are some suggestions for beginners. With these on hand, you will be well on your way to the best aromatherapy has to offer. (Note that I have used the common names here, but that there can be many different varieties of the same botanical species, each producing essential oils with somewhat different characteristics, properties, and therapeutic uses.)

Bergamot
   Description: citrusy-floral, clean, fresh, uplifting
   Uses: reduces anxiety, stress, depression; balances nervous tension; helps urinary tract infections; good for oily skin
   Blends well with: lavender, rose, patchouli
Cedarwood
   Description: soothing, soft, woody
   Uses: anger, aggression, bronchitis
   Blends well with: bergamot, jasmine, neroli, juniper, clary sage, rose
Chamomile
   Description: calming, soothing
   Uses: reduces stress, tension, anger, and anxiety; promotes restful sleep; healing to the skin, especially dry, itchy, inflamed or sunburned
   Blends well with: clary sage, neroli
Clary Sage
   Description: warm, spicy scent; relaxing, euphoric

Uses: relieves anxiety, tension, stress; promotes sense of well-being

Blends well with: citrus oils, sandalwood, lavender

Eucalyptus

Description: fresh, cooling, invigorating, stimulating

Uses: fights depression, exhaustion; brings about alertness; eases congestion from respiratory and sinus infections, coughs, colds; soothes tired muscles; brings down a fever

Blends well with: peppermint

Geranium

Description: flowery, roselike, calming (in small amounts), stimulating (in large amounts), balancing

Uses: reduces stress, depression, nervous tension, symptoms of PMS, fear; healing for skin disorders; bug repellent

Blends well with: lavender, bergamot, lemon, rosemary

Jasmine

Description: warm, floral, soothing

Uses: relieves depression, anxiety; mood uplifting; aphrodisiac; healing to damaged skin; good for abdomen during pregnancy

Blends well with: sandalwood

Lavender

Description: clean, fresh, floral, calming, gentle

Uses: reduces stress, nervous tension, anxiety; mood uplifting; helps insomnia and headaches; heals bruises, burns, damaged skin, insect bites

Blends well with: most oils, especially citrus oils, peppermint, eucalyptus

Lemon

Description: refreshing, uplifting, rejuvenating, cleansing

Uses: eases depression, tension; heightens mental alertness

Blends well with: other citrus oils, ylang-ylang

Neroli/Orange Blossom

Description: bittersweet, soothing, relaxing, uplifting

Uses: relieves stress, depression, anxiety, nervous tension, insomnia; instills confidence

Blends well with: sandalwood, jasmine

Peppermint

Description: refreshing, stimulating

Uses: increases alertness, relieves pain, indigestion, nausea, headaches; clears sinus congestion; combats fatigue

Blends well with: lavender, eucalyptus

Rose

Description: uplifting

Uses: regulates menstrual cycle, fights depression, treats frigidity, skin care

Blends well with: neroli, sandalwood, jasmine, lavender

Rosemary

Description: warm, spicy

Uses: promotes mental clarity and alertness; aids memory and concentration; eases muscle aches

Blends well with: frankincense, lavender, peppermint, cedarwood, cinnamon, other spice oils

Sandalwood

Description: warm, spicy-woody, calming, balancing

Uses: nervous tension, depression, fear, stress

Blends well with: ylang-ylang, rose, jasmine, lemon, benzoin, frankincense

Tea Tree

Description: spicy, strong, fresh

Uses: infections, acne, athlete's foot, herpes, first aid for cuts and abrasions

Blends well with: lavandin, lavender, clary sage, rosemary, pine, geranium, clove
(Note: Nothing will really mask tea tree's strong medicinal smell.)

Ylang-ylang

Description: sweet, soft, floral-spicy, heady, soothing
Uses: acne, high blood pressure, depression, impotence, stress; aphrodisiac
Blends well with: rosewood, jasmine, vetiver, bergamot, mimosa, rose, tuberose

Aromatherapy Blends with Carrier Oils

As mentioned previously, to make the most of your essential oils, you will also need to have some good quality carrier or base oils on hand. Since essential oils are so concentrated and strong, most cannot be applied directly to your skin (with the exception of lavender and possibly tea tree); they must be diluted in another oil base. These oils, generally cold-pressed vegetable oils, are referred to as carriers because they actually carry the essential oil and allow it to be used in various ways on the body. Among the most widely used are sweet almond, jojoba, and grapeseed oil. The most common application for using a carrier oil is in a massage or skin oil. Here is a recipe for an excellent carrier oil blend:

Professional Blend

This blend, according to Elly Jesser-Yellin, a certified aromatherapist at Beyond the Crescent Moon, a store in Great Neck, New York, which specializes in aromatherapy and perfumery, is good for at least 90 percent of all the formulas you will need.

Cleaning Bottles

Soap and hot water followed by distilled water rinses is a good way to wash out bottles after use. If some sticky organic material must be removed (e.g., resinified oils), a solvent such as essential oil of orange should probably work, followed by removal with warm, sudsy water. Rubbing alcohol is often recommended, but it contains quite a bit of water, which helps to slow down its already slow evaporation rate. If you decide to use denatured ethanol, make sure that it is denatured with wood alcohol (methanol), and see to it that it does not contain a bittering agent, since some of the denaturants are poison, and a bittering agent will remain behind after the alcohol has evaporated. This could contaminate the otherwise clean bottle. For best results, dry the alcohol on a glass plate; if it leaves a film behind, don't use it.

A Word about Diffusers

Diffusers are a convenient way to disperse the aroma of essential oils into the air. Here is some basic information.

Porcelain or Clay Pot

To use these diffusers, essential oils are mixed with water, while a candle is burned below, heating the water. The heat diffuses the aroma into the air.

Electric

The cost is about $40 to $100 depending on the brand. Follow the manufacturer's instructions, which usually say not to use any water (but some experts advise using a drop of water so you don't get a burnt smell).

Scent Ring

Add a few drops of essential oil to a ceramic glazed scent ring and place it on a lightbulb. The heat will diffuse the scent. (Note: I have not heard one good thing about scent rings. Even the experts agree that they pose a hazard since they often slip off the lightbulb or can catch fire if too much of the highly flammable essential oils get on the heated bulb. They are meant to be used by putting them on a cool lightbulb and the reservoir filled before turning on the light. Please use lightbulb rings with caution.)

A Basic Travel Kit

Here are some suggestions for a travel-ready aromatherapy kit.

Lavender: If you could travel with only one essential oil, it should be lavender. It's good for burns, cuts, sunburn pain, nausea, headaches, wounds, calming for nerves, and good in a bath to wind down jet lag.

Peppermint: It's helpful for headaches when inhaled, it is energizing when you need a lift, and it's good to get rid of the smell of cigarette smoke.

Eucalyptus: In case you catch a cold, have eucalyptus on hand.

In addition, take along at least one oil with a fragrance you really like—maybe geranium, sandalwood, ylang-ylang, rose—the choice is yours. Be careful with citrus oils, especially bergamot, if you'll be in the sun, as they can be phototoxic. If you can't take a diffuser or simmer pot with you on your trip, tissues or cotton balls will suffice, at least for those oils for which an inhalation is called for.

A hydrosol is a great product to take along, too. A hydrosol is sometimes called floral water—not just the kind where a few drops of oil are added to water, but a true hydrosol, a by-product of the actual plant. Rose or lavender are good choices. You can mist it onto your face during the flight to refresh and rehydrate your skin, it can calm your nerves, freshen air in a stuffy hotel room, soothe sunburned skin, and you can spray it onto your pillow or sheets for a pleasant night's sleep in a strange bed.

Safety Tips for Using Essential Oils

- Never leave candles burning without watching them, especially if you're very sleepy or sick.
- Don't put candles directly on furniture.
- Make sure flame is not near curtains or bedding.
- Don't get flame near oil, as essential oils are highly flammable substances.
- Don't leave a candle diffuser on without water.
- Be careful if using a lightbulb ring. These rings have been known to slip off the bulbs. Also, essential oils are highly flammable. Do not put oils directly on a hot lightbulb.
- Be careful when using essential oils in the bathtub. Many can burn or irritate the skin if not properly diluted. Also, the tub can become very slippery, especially if the essential oils are diluted in a carrier oil. Use caution when getting in and out of the tub.
- Do not ingest oils unless prescribed by a licensed, medically trained aromatherapist. Even then, many experts believe that essential oils should never be taken orally.

- Do patch tests on your skin before using an unfamiliar oil, especially if you have sensitive or allergic skin.
- Check if an oil you are planning to use is toxic and/or phototoxic.
- Check for warnings regarding toxicity, pregnancy, diabetes, epilepsy, skin sensitivity, and high or low blood pressure.
- If you suffer from asthma, do not use steam inhalation.
- Do not get the oils in your eyes. Although you won't do permanent damage, it will sting like crazy. If you do get the oils in your eyes, flushing them with water will only make the condition worse, because the water will disperse the oil even further. Instead, use vegetable oil, which will dilute the essential oil. Then flush the eye out with water.

CHAPTER 3

Encyclopedia of Essential Oils

Although there are hundreds of essential oils that can be produced from plants, the following are among the most commonly used for the majority of aromatherapy treatments. Each listing details how the oil is extracted, where the plant comes from, how the oil is commonly used, a history or traditional use of the oil (where appropriate), some other oils each mixes well with, and any precautions that should be taken when using these oils in aromatherapy treatments. Note that only lavender and possibly tea tree should be used undiluted (or neat) on the skin.

In addition to the common names listed here, the botanical name is also provided. Note, however, that there can be many different varieties of the same botanical species, each producing essential oils with somewhat different characteristics, properties, and therapeutic uses. There are several comprehensive books on the market that go into these differences in more detail. I recommend Julia Lawless's *The Illustrated Encyclopedia of Essential Oils: The*

Complete Guide to the Use of Oils in Aromatherapy and Herbalism.

If an oil is listed with an asterisk (*) next to its name, it is one of the most common being used in aromatherapy treatments today.

Angelica *(Angelica archangelica)*

The oil of this tall plant, grown in Eastern Europe, is derived by water distillation from its dried or fresh roots. Its scent is strong, spicy, and earthy in tone. Its greatest claim is that it builds physical and emotional stamina. It can also relieve nausea, strengthen the immune system, and alleviate feelings of anxiety and hopelessness. To treat congestion, colds, and respiratory problems, use two or three drops in a diffuser or aroma lamp three times per day, especially during the winter cold and flu season, either alone or in combination with eucalyptus and/or lemon essential oil, or it can be used in a salve. When used in a massage oil or bath, angelica also improves blood circulation and promotes general well-being.

In the Middle Ages, physicians used angelica to protect themselves from deadly infection, and it was also used in many secret remedies for a prolonged life. Because of its antiseptic, fungicidal, and antibacterial properties, it is still used as a treatment for wounds, infections, and skin fungus.

Recommended use: To ward off flu-season viruses, add a few drops of angelica essential oil to a diffuser, either on its own or in combination with lemon or eucalyptus oil.

Blends well with: bergamot, clary sage, eucalyptus, lemon, lemongrass, pine, juniper, and tea tree.

Caution: Angelica oil derived from the root is phototoxic

and can cause skin irritation when exposed to the sun. Avoid during pregnancy or if you suffer from diabetes.

Aniseed *(Pimpinella anisum)*

Aniseed oil has a sweet, fresh scent, and it is steam distilled from the seeds of the anise plant, which is cultivated mainly in India and China. Aniseed has long been used as a digestive aid and can be used to treat cramping, indigestion, or other digestive problems, including flatulence, which is especially valuable when the digestive difficulty is a result of nervous anxiety. It is also useful to treat spasmodic coughs, as aniseed oil is a good expectorant. Aniseed can promote a relaxing sleep. Aniseed, however, has a relatively high level of toxicity, so it is rarely used in aromatherapy treatments. Taken over long periods of time, it can become addictive, and it can slow circulation and possibly lead to brain damage.

Recommended use: For stomach cramps caused by nerves or tension, try a massage oil blend of one tablespoon of sweet almond oil combined with four or five drops of aniseed essential oil.

Blends well with: caraway, fennel, coriander.
   Caution: Do not take internally. Avoid during pregnancy. Due to its toxic levels, you're better off using alternative oils. Its principal constituent, anethole, is a known cause of dermatitis, so it is advisable to avoid contact with the skin, especially in those who are prone to allergic skin conditions.

Balm

See **Melissa.**

Basil or Sweet Basil *(Ocimum basilicum)*

This oil, which has a sweet licorice-like aroma, is extracted by steam-distillation of the flowering plant. The basil plant is native to Asia but now grows in Europe and North Africa. This herb is considered sacred in India and is a main ingredient in traditional Aryuvedic medicine.

It is a cheering oil and can be used to relieve stress, anxiety, nervousness, mental fatigue, and depression. It can help refresh the mind, especially when tired, and can increase concentration. Basil oil is also antiseptic, a digestive tonic, and a stimulant of hormones produced by the adrenal glands. It is useful for treating chronic colds, influenza, bronchitis, earache, epilepsy, fainting, fevers, gout, hiccups, hysteria, insomnia, migraine, paralysis, respiratory problems, nausea and vomiting, and whooping cough. It is believed to invigorate the body and spirit. Basil oil is also a useful insect repellent. The name *basil* has its origins in the Greek *basilicon,* which means a royal ointment.

Recommended use: Inhale directly from the bottle or place a drop or two on a cotton ball and inhale the aroma to refresh your mind and to increase mental alertness.

Blends well with: lavender, hyssop, bergamot, and clary sage.

Caution: Do not use basil essential oil internally. This essential oil is potentially toxic. Always avoid during pregnancy, as it stimulates menstruation. Use basil oil sparingly, as it can be a skin irritant, especially for people with sensitive skin.

Bay or Bay Leaf *(Pimenta racemosa)*

Essential oil of bay is extracted by water or steam-distillation from the leaves of the bay tree. Bay has its origins in Europe and the Americas, and the oil is currently produced in Dominica. The leaves from the bay tree were used for hundreds of years in European cooking. At the turn of the century, bay rum, a mixture of essential oil of bay and alcohol, was a popular hair tonic among English gentlemen. Today, bay oil is still considered useful as a scalp stimulant, hair rinse for dandruff sufferers, and to combat greasy hair.

This uplifting oil is a good tonic for respiratory ailments and infectious diseases, including lung conditions, colds, flu, and for opening up bronchial passages. It is also an antidepressant. Among its other benefits, bay can be used to heal brittle nails, rheumatism, poor circulation, and sprains. It has antiseptic, tonic, analgesic, and decongestant properties.

Recommended use: For colds, combine a few drops of bay leaf oil with eucalyptus and inhale or use in a diffuser.

Blends well with: citrus oils, spice oils, eucalyptus, lavender, lavandin, rosemary, geranium, and ylang-ylang.
   Caution: Can be irritating to the skin.

Benzoin or Styrax *(Styrax benzoin)*

Benzoin oil is not a pure essential oil but a resin, so it has to be warmed over hot water prior to use. It is extracted from the resin of a tree that is grown in Asia and has a sweet vanilla-like aroma. Benzoin might be familiar to some in the form of friar's balsam. It has been used for thousands of years to make incense and to get rid of lurking evil spirits. It is both soothing and stimulating. Inhale it to give yourself a boost of energy, as benzoin is said to revitalize a tired body. To treat depression, anger, and anxiety, benzoin is great in a massage oil, particularly when used around the neck and shoulder area. It calms the mind and the emotions. It is also good for stomach pain and for treating urinary tract infections. Benzoin is helpful for treating coughs, colds, and flu, especially when used in a steam inhalation. It can also be used externally to relieve cuts; dry, chapped, itchy skin; or dermatitis. For achy joints or arthritis, try benzoin in a carrier oil and massage it into the affected area or use it on a compress. Benzoin is a nice addition to a bath or, as in its traditional use, as an incense. Its main therapeutic benefits are as an antidepressant, anti-inflammatory, antiseptic, expectorant, and sedative oil. It is also a natural deodorant and preservative, useful in many recipes as such. The folk tradition of benzoin is that it can be used to encourage confidence and empowerment.

Recommended use: Put several drops of benzoin essential oil in a diffuser to treat respiratory problems, such as coughs, bronchitis, and asthma.

Blends well with: sandalwood, rose, jasmine, frankincense, myrrh, cypress, juniper, lemon, coriander, and with other spice oils.

   Caution: Benzoin oil can cause skin irritation in some people.

*Bergamot *(Citrus bergamia)*

This relaxing and refreshing oil comes from the bergamot tree, which is grown in Italy and Africa, and is part of the citrus family. The balancing oil is extracted by expression of the peel of the fruit and has a sweet, light, citrus fragrance that uplifts the spirit. Most people recognize this scent as that of Earl Grey tea. Bergamot has a definite calming effect; use it to treat stress, anxiety, everyday tension, or mental fatigue. It is, in fact, one of the most widely known oils for treating depression. It is named for the town of Bergamot, Italy, where it was originally sold. It remains one of the most common ingredients in eau de cologne.

Inhale the aroma before bedtime and you can expect to sleep peacefully. Bergamot oil is also a powerful antiseptic useful for treating cold sores, eczema, psoriasis, oily and blemished skin, and other skin conditions. Among its many uses, bergamot oil is especially beneficial for treating infections of the mouth, skin, respiratory system, and urinary tract, as well as halitosis and sore throats. It's great when used in a vaporizer to rid your home of unpleasant odors. This is a great oil to have with you when traveling to rid your hotel room of musty smells. Bergamot is also considered an appetite stimulant. It has been used to treat insect bites, as well as being an insect repellent.

Recommended use: Use several drops of bergamot essential oil in a diffuser to clear a musty room or add about twenty-five drops to a sixteen-ounce spray bottle filled with water. Spritz around the house for a clean-smelling environment.

Blends well with: geranium, chamomile, violet, coriander, lavender, neroli, patchouli, and rose.

Caution: To treat eczema, you would apply the bergamot to the skin. You *must,* however, dilute this essential oil, approximately 0.5 to 1 percent with a base oil. Undiluted on the skin, it can cause rather serious burns. Also, bergamot is phototoxic, due to a constituent called bergaptene, so it increases the skin's sun sensitivity. Used improperly, it can cause overpigmentation and, in worst-case scenarios, can lead to malignant melanomas. Never use bergamot on the skin in sunny weather. A bergaptene-free oil is available. Your best bet when dealing with bergamot is to see a professional aromatherapist.

Birch, White *(Betula alba)*

White birch oil is steam-distilled from the leaf buds of this tree found in such varied places as Eastern Europe, Russia, Germany, China, and Japan. It has a woody, balsamic aroma. Its primary aromatherapy use is in hair care products, including tonics and shampoos. It also is well-known for its benefits to the skin, and in the treatment of backaches, rheumatism, and arthritic conditions, due to its excellent anti-inflammatory and antiseptic properties.

Recommended use: Dilute white birch essential oil in a massage oil blend to treat sore, achy muscles.

Blends well with: other woody or balsamic essential oils.
    Caution: Do not confuse white birch *(Betula alba)* with sweet birch *(Betula lenta),* which, when absorbed through the skin, is a potentially toxic, hazardous substance.

Black Pepper or Pepper *(Piper nigrum)*

Unlike black pepper in its powdered herb form (the way most of us use pepper), the essential oil will not make you sneeze if you quickly inhale its aroma directly from the bottle. Black pepper essential oil is extracted by steam-distillation from the dried, crushed black peppercorns. It has a warm, spicy, pungent fragrance and is used as a stimulant and as a toning agent. Black pepper's aromatic powers are useful to combat tiredness, to sharpen mental alertness, and to energize the physical body. Black pepper is a particularly good scent to have on hand to help you stay awake when driving late at night; better, some would say, than a mug of strong, black coffee. Black pepper is a warming oil that is especially great to use during the cold winter months. It is wonderful for use in a massage oil for the abdomen and for aching muscles. It is often used in presports or dance rubs, as black pepper essential oil helps to maintain suppleness. It can also be used to treat arthritis, rheumatic pain, sprains, and joint stiffness. Among its other benefits, it can help relieve digestive disorders, such as constipation, diarrhea, flatulence, and nausea. Not everyone likes black pepper, but if you do, it really makes a statement.

Recommended use: Use a very small amount of black pepper oil in massage oil blends to help relieve muscular pain and stiffness. (Marathon runners sometimes use black pepper and rosemary before running.)

Blends well with: rosemary, sandalwood, frankincense, marjoram, and lavender.

Caution: Black pepper should be used in small quantities only. It can be irritating to the skin. Black pepper is contraindicated with homeopathic remedies.

Cajeput *(Melaleuca leucadendron)*

Cajeput oil is steam-distilled from the leaves and buds of the tree known as *Melaleuca leucadendron,* which grows in the Philippines, Malaysia, the Moluccas, Australia, and India. The tree, which has a white-colored bark, gets its name from the Malaysian term for *white tree, caju-puti.* This stimulating and antiseptic oil, which has a somewhat medicinal smell, improves mood and increases resistance to infections. It can be used to treat lung congestion. Cajeput is considered a good oil to help you unwind. It can be used in steam inhalation to clear nasal passages, but not before bedtime as its stimulating properties will keep you awake. Its use as a painkiller is effective to relieve the symptoms of sore throats and headaches. It is also known to be a powerful reliever of toothache pain, but it should be diluted in a carrier oil before it is applied to the tooth area (10 percent essential oil in the mixture). It is also a well-known remedy for sore muscles, and it can be used for treating oily skin and acne.

Recommended use: For colds and flu, use cajeput essential oil in a steam inhalation to clear nasal passages.

Blends well with: eucalyptus, juniper, and mint.
  Caution: Can be irritating to the skin.

Camphor *(Cinnamomum camphora)*

Camphor essential oil is steam-distilled from the wood and leaves of camphor trees that are at least half a century old. These trees are grown mainly in China, Japan, India, Ceylon, and Madagascar. Its fragrance is similar to the medicinal smell of eucalyptus. Long ago, camphor was worn around the neck to ward off infection. Most of us associate camphor's smell with mothballs, but that well-known scent is synthetic, and the vapors can be dangerous. White camphor essential oil, however, is much safer and can be used to treat such ailments as the common cold and to care for oily and pimply skin. Skip the cold shower and take a sniff or two of some camphor oil to turn off sexual feelings. It can also be used as an insect repellent.

Recommended uses: To help relieve cold feet, add six to eight drops of camphor essential oil to a footbath. Use about twenty drops in an aroma lamp as an insect repellent. For a cleansing facial, add two drops of camphor oil combined with four drops of juniper and four drops of peppermint to a bowl of steaming (not boiling water.) Place a towel over your head and inhale the steam for about seven to eight minutes.

Blends well with: juniper, lemon, lime, and angelica.

Caution: Use sparingly. Prolonged inhalation will cause headaches, so just open the bottle, take a quick whiff, and close it back up. Those suffering from epilepsy should completely avoid camphor. Do not use it with children under five years old. Use it in moderation externally, as camphor oil can be irritating to sensitive skin. Camphor essential oil is contraindicated with homeopathic remedies.

Cardamom (*Elettaria cardamomum*)

This expensive essential oil is steam-distilled from the seeds of a plant that is closely related to ginger. Its fragrance is sweet, spicy, and warming, and it is produced in such areas as India, Ceylon, Guatemala, El Salvador, China, and the Middle East. The early Egyptians used cardamom as a perfume and incense.

This oil can be used to help with digestive problems, including nausea, flatulence, and diarrhea. It is a known tonic and is great when used in a light, invigorating bath oil.

Recommended use: For a stimulating bath, use in a bath blend with other oils.

Blends well with: rose, frankincense, orange, bergamot, cinnamon, ylang-ylang, cedarwood, and neroli.

Caution: Cardamom oil might be a skin irritant to those with sensitive skin.

Carrot Seed *(Daucus carota)*

Produced mainly in France, carrot seed essential oil is extracted by steam-distillation from the dried fruit or ground seeds. It has a similar fragrance to carrots: sweet, earthy, and fruity. It aids in digestive disorders and to promote menstruation. It can also be used to treat such skin conditions as dermatitis, eczema, psoriasis, rashes, and sunburn. It is considered to be especially beneficial for older skin, as it can restore the skin's elasticity and possibly even reduce wrinkles, but it should not be used on oily skin types or to treat acne. It makes an excellent skin care blend when used with sweet almond oil as a carrier.

Aside from its benefits to the skin and hair, this oil is considered a stimulant to endocrine function. It is thought to stimulate the lymph system and to aid in women's milk production after childbirth.

Recommended use: For sunburn relief, mix five drops of carrot seed oil with fifteen drops of lavender oil. Blend into two ounces of aloe vera oil and apply to the affected skin.

Blends well with: cedarwood, geranium, and most citrus essential oils.

Caution: Do not use during pregnancy.

*Cedar, Cedarwood, or Atlas Cedar *(Cedrus atlantica)*

Essential oil of cedarwood is extracted by steam-distillation of wood chips and sawdust from the bark. Cedarwood, with its woody aroma, is believed to have life-giving and calming effects, especially the oil of cedar trees from Morocco and Algeria. The tree also grows in America, Lebanon, southern Europe, and Asia. Some say that cedarwood oil may have been the first essence to be extracted from a plant. It is one of the most ancient aromatics, used during religious ceremonies in ancient Egypt. The early Egyptians used a primitive distilling method to produce cedarwood gum for their mummification process. They also used it as an insect repellent, for which it is still used today. Atlas cedar is believed to have been used extensively by the Egyptians, in fact, in perfumes and cosmetics. Through the centuries, it became apparent that cedar had tremendous healing properties as well.

Cedarwood is considered a deeply relaxing, harmonizing, and spiritually strengthening oil. It is good for relieving stress and nervous tension. Cedarwood is known to eliminate blockages and toxins—physically, mentally, and emotionally. It cleanses and purifies the body, the skin, and the environment. As an inhalant, it can benefit the bronchial system, is an expectorant to relieve coughing, and an antiseptic for mucusy coughs and colds. Cedarwood is also a diuretic with healing antiseptic properties to aid in treating urinary and kidney infections. It is an astringent and is considered healing for the skin and scalp, and it is used for skin rashes and conditions such as eczema, acne, and oily skin. It also controls oily hair, dandruff, and hair loss, and is used as a tonic for the glandular and nervous systems. Cedar is reportedly an aphrodisiac, encouraging sexual feelings. Some say it even helps in the fight against cellulite. Its warm, woody scent makes this a great room fragrance, too. Even use it in your closet as a moth repellent. In Tibet, cedarwood is used as a temple incense.

Recommended use: To treat bronchial problems, add a few drops to a simmer pot or diffuser.

Blends well with: lemon, rose, bergamot, jasmine, neroli, juniper, hyssop, sandalwood, patchouli, rosemary, and clary sage.

Caution: Avoid during pregnancy. Also, there are several trees that produce essential oils, but only use the oil from the atlas cedar *(Cedrus atlantica)* for aromatherapy purposes.

*Chamomile: Roman Chamomile *(Anthemis noblis)* and German or Blue Chamomile *(Matricaria chamomilla)*

Roman chamomile is extracted by steam-distillation from the flowers and leaves of the plant; German or blue chamomile is extracted by steam-distillation from the flowers. Whichever you choose, chamomile is well known as having a soothing effect on both mind and body. Roman chamomile comes from Southern and Eastern Europe, and German or blue chamomile, as one would expect, is a native of Germany, although it is cultivated in Hungary, Russia, Egypt, and parts of North America. Chamomile contains azulene, which has great healing and antibacterial qualities. German chamomile has a greater azulene content, giving it its more characteristic blue color. It is generally more expensive than Roman chamomile and has a stronger spicy-green aroma, but both have very similar healing benefits. Most people do not recognize the powerful scent of chamomile essential oil the first time they smell it. It is quite different from the soothing chamomile tea smell most of us know.

It can help with stomach and intestinal problems and cramps. It is particularly helpful for treating skin irritations, rashes, abscesses, acne, eczema, and hives. Chamomile also strengthens tissue, cleanses the skin, and protects dry skin, and it has been used for centuries to highlight and condition hair.

All chamomile oil is gentle, suitable for the young and old alike, but German chamomile is one of the few essential oils that can be used on inflamed skin. Try using it on a cotton compress. Soak a compress in hot water with a few drops of chamomile to relieve severe cramps. Add a few drops to a warm bath to relieve the itchiness of many types of skin allergies, dermatitis, eczema, or psoriasis. Chamomile essential oil can be used, also, to care for a bee sting. It is one of the best oils to use to ease anger, anxiety, and tension; it also helps relieve insomnia, headaches, and menstrual disorders.

Chamomile is anti-inflammatory, antispasmodic, and a nerve sedative. In ancient Egypt, chamomile was dedicated to the sun due to its fever-reducing powers. Today, it is still a great oil to use in a diffuser or bath: Breathe in the calming fragrance. German or blue chamomile is particularly useful for sufferers of high blood pressure and to treat shingles. Roman chamomile is a good oil to use during pollen season.

Recommended uses: Use Roman chamomile in an aroma lamp or diffuser to relieve allergies. For a relaxing bath, use ten drops of Roman chamomile, three drops of lavender, two drops of tangerine, and two drops of geranium. Blend the essential oils into 1¾ ounces of carrier oil, such as hazelnut oil, and add the mixture to a warm bath. This is an especially good blend to use during pregnancy.

Blends well with: rose, cedar, clary sage, bergamot, neroli, lavender, and geranium.

Cinnamon *(Cinnamomum zeylanicum)*

The cinnamon essential oil is extracted from two different parts of a tree that is a member of the laurel family and that grows in China and Ceylon. Cinnamon bark oil is steam-distilled from the woody portion (bark). Cinnamon leaf oil is produced from the leaves or twigs. Cinnamon is one of the world's oldest aromatic plants, even garnering mention in the Old Testament.

This sweet, warm, spicy, and stimulating oil can be used to treat stress, anxiety, tension, or mental fatigue. It is a strong antiseptic and has a cleansing effect, so it is highly valuable in combating infections and contagious diseases. It is good for colds, flu, headache, toothache, and sore muscles. Cinnamon oil is also known as a circulatory, heart, digestive, and respiratory stimulant. It is a very comforting oil, especially nice during the cold weather. It makes a delicious room fragrance, one that reminds many of Christmas. Some research has shown that most men find cinnamon to be irresistible, maybe because it reminds them of the love and comfort of cookies baking in the kitchen. It is considered an aphrodisiac, so it is sometimes used to treat impotence. It is also antispasmodic and an antivenom agent (it can be used to treat snakebites). Cinnamon is supposed to diffuse hostile energy. This is a great scent to fill your home with if you're trying to sell your house. Real estate agents know that it's easier to make a sale when the house smells like home. If you don't have the essential oil, cinnamon tea bags in water on the stove is a pleasant alternative.

Recommended uses: For a great room spray, especially during the winter holidays, try two drops of cinnamon essential oil combined with ten drops of pine. Add this to a spray bottle filled with water and spray your carpeting. You can also use the blend in a diffuser or simmer pot. Another wonderful room scent is a combination of cinnamon and sweet orange. Use it in a diffuser or simmer pot.

Blends well with: ylang-ylang, sandalwood, lime, sweet orange, pine, juniper, and jasmine.

   Caution: Cinnamon bark oil can cause skin sensitization; do not use it on the skin. Use cinnamon oil in small amounts.

Citronella *(Cymbopogon nardus)*

Citronella essential oil is extracted by steam-distillation from a grass that is found in South America, China, and Indonesia. This light, warm, woody, fresh oil has a strong, lemon scent that some say is uplifting, as well as being a natural deodorizer. It is believed to encourage self-expression and creativity, so it is considered a good oil for actors and writers. It can be used as an insect and cat repellent, but it is not often used in aromatherapy treatments. It is a frequent ingredient in many commercially produced soaps and household disinfectants.

Recommended use: As an outdoor insect repellent, place a drop of the essential oil onto a lightbulb *before* you turn it on. Do not put oil on a hot lightbulb. As the bulb heats up, the aroma will be diffused into the general area.

Blends well with: lemon, geranium, bergamot, orange, cedarwood, and pine.

   Caution: People with very sensitive skin, including sufferers of eczema and dermatitis, should avoid contact with this oil. Avoid during pregnancy.

*Clary Sage or Clary *(Salvia sclarea)*

Clary sage essential oil is steam-distilled from the flowers and flowering tops of the plant, which are in bloom from May through September. This unique, soothing oil with a warm, nutty, haylike aroma became popular in Europe in the sixteenth century. The plant from which clary sage essential oil is derived is native to Italy, Syria, and southern regions of France. Today it is mainly cultivated in France and Russia, but also in Yugoslavia and Spain. The oil varies greatly, depending on the conditions in which the plant is grown.

It is used to make eau de cologne and is considered a soothing aftershave, especially good for shaving over rashes and inflamed skin. It is known to be cell regenerating, is a muscle relaxant, and is generally helpful in relieving anxiety, stress, tension, anger, moodiness, and melancholy. For the workaholics among us, the inhalation of clary sage is a valuable aid to nervous exhaustion and work-related burnout. Clary is an uplifting oil; some describe its effect as euphoric, while others simply find it incredibly relaxing and warming, especially when they are dealing with outside stresses. It is supposed to inspire a sense of well-being to the spirit, boost self-confidence, and help break through emotional blockages.

While it has many of the properties of sage, it is used much more frequently in aromatherapy treatments, probably because it has a lower level of a substance found in sage (thujone), which in high doses, can be toxic.

Clary sage has been called clear eye and was used traditionally for healing eye conditions. A recognized aphrodisiac, clary is known as a passion arouser due to its sensual properties. Clary sage contains a hormonelike agent that is similar to estrogen that regulates hormonal balance, which makes it a good choice for premenstrual discomfort, relieving menopausal hot flashes, and according to some aromatherapists, as an aid for female frigidity. Some claim that clary sage essential oil induces dramatic and colorful dreams. It is also reported to be particularly helpful to those searching for a muse in their creative endeavors. It is recognized as an oil that brings out the unexpected.

Use it in a massage oil for the lower back and abdomen before and during menstruation to relieve cramping. It is also useful in massage to help with tired, sore, or injured muscles. Clary sage is also very useful in beauty and hair care products, as it is a good choice for oily hair and skin, dandruff, and wrinkles. Inhale the aroma or mix it into a carrier oil and rub it into the chest and throat area about three times a day to soothe a sore throat.

Recommended uses: For hair care, add a couple of drops to about ¼ ounce of your shampoo or conditioner. Use a few drops of clary sage oil in a bath oil blended with citrus oils, sandalwood, and lavender or with rose and lavender. (Clary, lavender, and rose is a good combination for PMS.)

Blends well with: jasmine, geranium, lavender, rose, sandalwood, cypress, and citrus oils.

Cautions: Avoid alcohol when using clary sage. Do not use clary sage to excess, as its benefits will be diminished and all you will get is a headache. Do not use it if you are taking medication containing iron. Avoid using clary sage during pregnancy.

Clove *(Eugenia caryophyllata)*

Clove oil is a strong oil that is extracted by steam-distillation from the cloves, or the unopened flower buds, of an evergreen tree that grows in India and Africa. A powerful antiseptic, clove has been used for its healing powers for centuries. Medically, clove has been useful in strengthening eyesight, as well as in the prevention of disease, infection, and to treat illness, due to its antibacterial, antiseptic, and analgesic properties. Traditionally, it has been good for treating oral infections and toothaches as it is very comforting when rubbed onto gums. According to some aromatherapists, clove oil is useful in mouthwashes and gargles. Clove is also used to treat digestive problems, muscular disorders, asthma, nausea, and sinusitis. This oil calms the emotions, so clove can also be used to treat stress, anxiety, tension, or mental fatigue. It is also used to sterilize surgical instruments, as a mosquito repellent, and as a room freshener.

Recommended use: To relieve toothache discomfort, add a drop of clove oil to a cotton ball. Apply to the aching tooth.

Blends well with: rose, lavender, clary sage, bergamot, ylang-ylang, and bay leaf.

Caution: Due to its strong nature, clove oil should always be diluted before applying it to your skin. Clove bud oil has been reported as a cause of some cases of skin sensitization. People with sensitive skin and those who suffer from eczema or dermatitis should avoid clove bud oil altogether. Avoid during pregnancy. Always use in moderation (less than a 1 percent dilution). Note: Clove has such a strong scent that it can overpower other scents in a blend.

Coriander *(Coriandum sativum)*

Coriander essential oil is extracted by steam-distillation of the dried fruit or seed of a plant that grows in the Far East,

North Africa, Spain, England, and Russia. It is from the same plant family as caraway, dill, and fennel.

The warm, sweet, spicy oil is an antispasmodic and can be used to treat stomach trouble, including flatulence and constipation. It is good as a massage blend to relieve stiff, achy muscles. It can also be used in a refreshing, stimulating bath. Coriander oil is useful for relief from painful menstruation. Coriander also has a relatively high estrogen content, perhaps explaining its eroticizing effect. Coriander is often used to flavor liqueurs, such as Chartreuse and Benedictine, and is also one of the main ingredients in lily of the valley perfumes.

Recommended use: Use four drops of coriander combined with four drops of neroli in a diffuser to stimulate creativity.

Blends well with: rose, jasmine, clary sage, petitgrain, geranium, orange, lemon, bergamot, sandalwood, ginger, and neroli.

Caution: Use in moderation as coriander can be stupefying if used in large doses. Avoid during pregnancy.

Cumin (Cuminum cyminum)

Cumin essential oil is extracted by steam-distillation of the seeds. Originally grown in Egypt, it can now be found in many Mediterranean areas. It has a warm, musky, spicy fragrance that can be compared to aniseed. Considered by some to be an erotic or aphrodisiac oil, cumin oil makes a wonderful addition for luxurious, sensuous baths, body lotions, or perfumes.

Other therapeutic uses include stimulating digestion, as an antispasmodic, and for reducing flatulence. Cumin is very similar to coriander in its properties and uses.

Recommended use: Add one or two drops of cumin to a warm bath, combined with lavender or other essential oils of your choice. Be sure to dilute it first in a carrier.

Blends well with: rose, cardamom, cinnamon, ylang-ylang, jasmine, lavender, rosemary, sandalwood, tonka bean, and patchouli.

Caution: Cumin essential oil can be phototoxic and can be irritating to skin when exposed to sunlight. It is also inadvisable to use large quantities of cumin in perfume. Avoid during pregnancy. Some suggest using coriander instead of cumin.

Cypress *(Cupressus sempervirens)*

Cypress oil has a smoky, woody aroma that refreshes, restores, and tones. It is extracted by steam-distillation from the leaves and twigs of the cypress tree, a southern European evergreen. Historically, the fragrance of cypress was a popular scent of the Assyrians.

Cypress oil is useful as a remedy to treat stress, anxiety, tension, or mental fatigue. Its astringent properties are good for blemishes and oily skin. It is also a natural deodorant and an antiperspirant that is good for sweaty feet when used in a footbath. Cypress oil can be beneficial in a massage oil for the abdominal area during menstruation. Also massage it on areas where there is cellulite or use it in a warm bath combined with juniper. Cypress is considered a good oil to use during menopause. It has restorative and antispasmodic properties, making it a good choice for treating asthma attacks. Just place a few drops on a tissue or handkerchief and inhale it when needed. Cypress oil can also be used to treat maladies ranging from coughs and influenza to rheumatism, wounds, and varicose veins. This oil is also a natural insect repellent. Cypress is an ancient symbol of comfort, so when in need of solace, try inhaling this aroma.

Recommended uses: For foot odor, soak feet in a warm bowl of water to which you have added five or six drops of cypress oil. Or, combine cypress oil with lemon oil to combat foot perspiration. For hemorrhoids, add five drops of cypress oil to a shallow bath or sitz bath. Mix well and soak.

Blends well with: benzoin, clary sage, cedarwood, sandalwood, lavender, marjoram, orange, lime, juniper, pine, bergamot, and lemon.

*Eucalyptus *(Eucalyptus globulus)*

Steam-distilled from the leaves of the eucalyptus tree (or gum tree), this familiar clean, fresh-smelling essential oil is used to treat stress, anxiety, tension, depression, and physical or mental exhaustion with its calming and relaxing properties. Its origin as a distilled oil dates back to at least 1788. Australian Aboriginies have used eucalyptus leaves to heal their wounds. It was brought to Europe in the late eighteenth century. Today it is cultivated not only in Australia, but in Egypt, Algeria, Spain, Portugal, India, South Africa, and the west coast of the United States.

An essential oil found in any basic kit, eucalyptus has numerous uses. While probably best known as an effective treatment against infections, respiratory difficulties, asthma, laryngitis, colds, stuffy noses, coughs, and sinusitis (think Vicks VapoRub), it can also be used in the treatment of urinary tract infections, cystitis, candida, diabetes, and sunburn. Blend eucalyptus essential oil in chest rubs or use it in a vaporizer in a sickroom to kill airborne germs. (People have actually moved to locations where any of the three hundred varieties of eucalyptus trees grow in order to improve their health.) Its most common use is probably in a steam inhalation to treat a cold or sinus problem. Eucalyptus oil is anti-inflammatory, antibiotic, diuretic, analgesic, soothing, and deodorizing. It is especially regarded as an excellent antiseptic. Some surgeons use eucalyptus to clean postoperative wounds. Eucalyptus can be used to cool emotions, aid concentration, and strengthen the immune system. It is great for tired, achy muscles or to cool down a fever. Eucalyptus is also beneficial for insect bites and stings, and is a known insect repellent. Combined with bergamot, it is very useful in treating shingles and cold sores. It helps acne and it will often clear up a pimple overnight.

Recommended uses: For sinusitis or bronchitis, inhale a drop or two of eucalyptus oil from a cotton ball or tissue when your nose is very stuffy, or put three to five drops into a diffuser pot to benefit the whole room, or put three drops on a hot, wet washcloth; hold the cloth over your face for three to four minutes every few hours; and keep your eyes closed. For pimples, apply a drop to a pimple using a cotton swab, and it just might clear up overnight.

Blends well with: lemon, verbena, lavender, pine, peppermint, thyme, rosemary, marjoram, bergamot, and cedarwood.

Caution: Eucalyptus is extremely toxic when taken internally. Eucalyptus is contraindicated with homeopathic medicines. Do not even store them near each other, as they can cancel out the other's benefits.

Fennel *(Foeniculum vulgare)*

The essential oil of sweet fennel is steam-distilled from the seeds, roots, and leaves. This essential oil has a sweet, aniseed-like aroma. Sweet fennel grows mainly in Europe, especially France, Italy, and Germany. Fennel was used to ward off evil spirits during medieval times. Fennel oil produces hormonal effects on women, due perhaps to the estrogen-like plant hormone that it contains. It is good for breast-feeding problems, including, some say, when used in a breast-firming massage oil and to promote milk production after childbirth. Long recognized for its value for the female reproductive system, fennel is also believed to regulate the menstrual cycle, reduce menstrual cramps, and alleviate the symptoms of premenstrual syndrome. It is also considered a helpful oil to use during menopause. A carminative, fennel can also be used to help with stomach trouble in combination with other essential oils that stimulate digestion. Fennel can be used to help control water retention when used in the bath, as well as alleviating nausea, vomiting, flatulence, and even hiccups. Fennel is a pleasant oil for use in skin care regimens and for use in a massage oil on areas where you have cellulite, where its anti-toxic properties really go to work. Fennel has also been used to combat alcohol poisoning and in the treatment of alcoholics during rehabilitation.

Recommended uses: For breast-feeding problems, use one drop of fennel oil in one teaspoon of olive oil. At night, rub this into the breasts after nursing. For hiccups, inhale neat from the bottle or use it in a steam inhalation.

Blends well with: geranium, lavender, rose, and sandalwood.

Caution: This essential oil can be hazardous, so use it sparingly. It can irritate skin. Never use it on children below age six. Avoid during pregnancy. Do not use fennel oil if you suffer from epilepsy.

Note: Sweet fennel (described above), should not be confused with bitter fennel, which should not be used in aromatherapy.

Frankincense or Olibanum *(Boswellia carteri)*

The essential oil (actually an incense) of frankincense is produced through steam-distillation of the oleo-gum-resin from a small tree that grows in North Africa. The gum is produced mainly in Somalia, East Africa. Its fragrance can be described as spicy, balsamic, and woody. It smells like incense, and, in fact, it has been used throughout history as such. It is a scent very familiar to many as a church smell.

In Biblical times, frankincense was considered one of the most precious substances known. It was, in fact, a significant commodity of ancient trade for both religious rites and for perfumes. It is a sedative and a skin tonic that may slow the wrinkling process. It can relieve anxiety and nervous tension, and it creates a spiritual atmosphere. According to Patricia Davis in *Aromatherapy: An A–Z*, "Frankincense has, among its physical properties, the ability to slow down and deepen the breath . . . which is very conducive to prayer and meditation." It is also excellent for toning and caring for dry and/or mature skin types. Many claim that frankincense has rejuvenating qualities. Ancient Egyptians actually used it in rejuvenation face masks. It is an antiseptic, blood coagulant, and is cleansing—psychically and otherwise. Frankincense is very useful for purifying polluted air.

Recommended uses: To get rid of the smell of smoke, diffuse frankincense into a room. You can use a simmer pot or burn the resin form of frankincense. These methods are also useful for creating an atmosphere suitable for meditation or for a Christmas party. A bath blend of frankincense and juniper is very relaxing after a stressful day. Create a facial oil for mature skin by combining ten drops of frankincense with ten drops of patchouli. The essential oils should be blended into two ounces of carrier oil (sweet almond or jojoba with 10 percent wheat germ oil). To treat wrinkles, use a blend of fifteen drops of frankincense and five drops of cypress oil in the carrier base.

Blends well with: rose, lavender, myrrh, patchouli, neroli, sandalwood, and juniper.

Garlic *(Allium sativum)*

The essential oil of garlic is extracted by steam-distillation of the fresh bulbs from this herb. Garlic is cultivated throughout the world and the oil is produced in such countries as France, China, and Japan. The oil has a strong, familiar odor, very similar to the garlic we are familiar with from cooking. Because of its telltale odor, garlic oil is not used in many aromatherapy home remedies. It is certainly not something you'd be inclined to use in a face cream or a perfume. While its more common form of late has been in garlic capsules, which are taken internally to reduce high blood pressure and as protection from heart disease, there are some skin benefits to using garlic essential oil externally. Due to its powerful healing properties—it is antiseptic, heals wounds, is a fungicide, and detoxifies—it is widely accepted as being quite beneficial in treating some medical problems. Its common uses include treating warts, calluses, and corns.

Recommended use: To treat warts or corns, apply one or two drops of garlic (undiluted) to the area once a day. Cover with a sterile cotton bandage. Repeat daily until healed, at which time, treat the area with wheat germ oil or with a mixture of vitamin E and lavender.

Caution: Garlic has been known to cause sensitization in some people.

*Geranium (Pelargonium graveolens)

This essential oil is distilled from the leaves and stem of the common plant, and is imported mainly from an island located in the West Indian Ocean. It has a fresh, leafy, floral-rose aroma that is very strong, but not really like the geraniums we are all familiar with. Geranium has been considered a healing plant throughout the centuries, especially for wounds and fractures.

It is best known as a balancing or regulating oil for the mind and body. Geranium is used to reduce stress, anxiety, tension, or mental fatigue. It is an antidepressant that helps balance the adrenal system and restores the stability of the emotions. Geranium, in fact, is thought to be rich in plant hormones, which can aid the body in regulating the human hormonal system. These hormonal balancing properties are believed to help with hypersensitivity and the many emotional symptoms associated with PMS. Geranium lifts the spirits, balances mood swings, and can invigorate you when you're feeling indifferent to the world.

The essential oil is great in helping to fight exhaustion after a long flight, and is used in preparations for cellulite, eczema, psoriasis, herpes, and shingles. It is a diuretic, benefits diabetes, and stimulates circulation. It is also an astringent oil that benefits all skin types. In fact, it is believed to strengthen the skin and improve elasticity. It can also be used in the treatment of such diverse ailments as frostbite and infertility. Geranium oil is sometimes used to treat menopausal bleeding. It is also used as an insect repellent.

Recommended uses: Blend geranium with rosemary and inhale this to aid with memory problems. Diffuse geranium with lemon and immortelle to fight off the craving to smoke. Use geranium with bergamot and lavender in a diffuser as a room freshener. Add geranium to a bath blend with bergamot and lavender to combat depression.

Blends well with: rosewood, lemon, bergamot, lavender, rose, and with any other floral oils.

Caution: People with very sensitive skin, including sufferers of eczema and dermatitis, should avoid contact with this oil, as it can sometimes cause allergic reactions.

Ginger *(Zinagiber officinalis)*

Ginger is described as a fiery, fortifying, and comforting essential oil, which is extracted by steam-distillation from the ground root. Its aroma is fresh, warm, and woody-spicy, and does not closely resemble the familiar aroma of dried ginger. Its origins are in Asia, but this spice was brought to Europe during the Middle Ages, making its way on the Spice Route.

It is great in a massage oil or in compresses for aching muscles or for pain from rheumatism. It is especially known for its curative properties for the digestive system, as an aid for nausea, constipation, cramps, indigestion, and loss of appetite. It can also be used to reduce stress, anxiety, tension, or mental fatigue. According to Jean Valnet in *The Practice of Aromatherapy*, women of Senegal wore belts made of gingerroot as a way to arouse their husbands.

Recommended use: A blend of ginger and orange essential oils are great for a warming bath on a cold winter day.

Blends well with: orange and other citrus oils.

Caution: Use in small dosages, since ginger oil can irritate the skin. People with very sensitive skin, including sufferers of eczema and dermatitis, should completely avoid contact with this oil.

Grapefruit *(Citrus paradisi)*

The essential oil of grapefruit is extracted by cold-pressing of the fresh peel. Not surprisingly, the oil is produced primarily in California. Known to refresh and uplift the spirit, grapefruit essential oil has a fresh, sweet, citrus aroma that helps combat nervous exhaustion, stress, depression, and moodiness. Some say it has a euphoric effect, producing a general feeling of well-being and renewed energy or a second wind. It also has an antiseptic and toning effect on skin and tissues, so it aids in relieving congested and oily skin, as well as acne. This is a good oil to use when treating cellulitis, as it is believed to help the body rid itself of dangerous toxins. It can have a positive effect on eating disorders, too, including anorexia and overeating, as it is believed to have a balancing effect on the appetite (remember the grapefruit diet?). It also stimulates the liver and gallbladder.

Recommended uses: For a wonderfully refreshing bath, two drops of grapefruit oil can be combined with three drops of bergamot and three drops of rosewood. Add this to a warm bath and soak for ten minutes. Grapefruit oil can also be used in a bath with other oils, such as lemon, juniper, and rosemary. Grapefruit oil in a diffuser is a sure way to lift the spirits.

Blends well with: bergamot, lemon, palmarosa, juniper, neroli, rosemary, cypress, lavender, rosewood, geranium, cardamom, as well as other spicy essential oils.

Caution: Do not use grapefruit oil on the skin in direct sunlight.

Hyssop *(Hyssopus officinalis)*

Hyssop oil is steam-distilled from the flowers or the whole plant. Mediterranean in origin, this sweet-spicy, camphor-like oil comes from a plant cultivated today in France, Italy, Spain, and Yugoslavia. Hyssop is an ancient herb that has been used throughout the centuries for its medicinal and romantic properties. The ancient Greeks and Hebrews considered hyssop essential oil sacred, as hyssop brooms were used to sweep sacred temples.

Hyssop can be used to treat stress, anxiety, tension, or mental fatigue. It contains warming properties and in addition to treating stress is believed to increase mental alertness and heighten spirituality. It is antiseptic in nature, as well as a tonic and decongestant. Hyssop oil can be used as an expectorant to treat colds and flu, and to help heal bruised skin. It is generally known for its beneficial uses in clearing up respiratory disorders, especially bronchitis, and in relieving the symptoms of hay fever. Use it in a diffuser or spray to protect rooms from infections. It can also be helpful in a massage oil, combined with oils such as sandalwood and lavender. This blend would also be beneficial in a diffuser.

Hyssop is not an oil commonly used by beginners, and it can be hard to find. It is best left to the professionals.

Recommended use: For relieving congestion and symptoms of bronchitis, add about three drops of hyssop to a simmer pot, together with six drops of lavender and six drops of sandalwood.

Mixes well with: clary sage, lavender, lemon, sage, rosemary, and sandalwood.

Caution: Do not use hyssop during pregnancy, as it is believed to stimulate menstruation. Do not use it if you are suffering from high blood pressure or epilepsy, as it can set off a seizure in those prone to them.

Immortelle, Helichrysum, or Everlast (*Helichrysum angustifolium*)

This essential oil, which is extracted by steam-distillation from the fresh flowers in full bloom, has a sweet, honeylike aroma. This evergreen herb grows wild throughout the Mediterranean. It is said that this oil lets you look within yourself and achieve self-awareness.

Immortelle is particularly useful in treating disorders and allergies of the skin, lymphatic system, and mucous membranes, especially illnesses related to environmental irritants. Allergy-related rashes and eczema are often treated with immortelle in conjunction with lavender and rockrose. It also works well in combination with angelica for the treatment of allergies, and with lemon and geranium to help quit the smoking habit. It is anti-inflammatory, fungicidal, and astringent, and can be used to provide relief from burns and dry, chapped skin. Immortelle is also considered an oil that helps to rejuvenate cells. This oil can be used successfully in a diffuser or aroma lamp, bath, or diluted in a base oil.

Recommended use: To treat inflamed abscesses, combine immortelle with lavender (about fifteen drops in total). For a mildly inflamed abscess, add essential oils to two pints of boiled hot water and treat the wound with a hot compress. For a severely inflamed abscess, add oils to two pints of cold water and treat the area with a cold compress. (Note: If the condition does not improve, seek medical attention.)

Blends well with: angelica, grapefruit, bergamot, lavender, verbena, orange, neroli, and cypress.

*Jasmine *(Jasminum officinale)* or Jasmine Absolute *(Jasminum grandiflorum)*

Jasmine essential oil is extracted with solvents from the flowers of the jasmine bush, which is a member of the olive family. This warm, exotic, floral scent is originally from East India. Today, it is cultivated in southern France, Morocco, Algeria, China, and Egypt. It relaxes, soothes, promotes self-confidence and optimism, deepens moods, and reputedly opens one up to sensual love.

It is an excellent oil for alleviating depression, nervous exhaustion, and stress-related ailments, including skin allergies, dermatitis, and eczema. Used throughout the ages as a powerful aphrodisiac, jasmine absolute has been used to treat impotence and frigidity with its soothing and relaxing effects. It is wonderful if used in an aroma lamp or diffuser, bath, or lotion, but it should never be taken internally.

For skin care, it is beneficial for dry, greasy, irritated, and sensitive skin, but it is good for all skin types. Jasmine oil is useful to treat muscular spasms and respiratory ailments such as catarrh, coughs, hoarseness, and laryngitis. It also is used to relieve labor pains and uterine disorders.

Jasmine is one of the more expensive essential oils available since a large number of blossoms, which have to be gathered at night when their scent is at their peak, are needed to produce even a few drops of this oil. But you can get more for your money if you use it sparingly with a diffuser or put a drop on a tissue or handkerchief and inhale the scent. You only need a very small quantity to benefit from its exquisite power. A drop can even be applied directly to the body.

It has earned its reputation as the king of flower oils. In India, the jasmine plant is referred to as "queen of the night" or "moonshine in the garden." Rumor has it that Cleopatra seduced Mark Antony by wearing jasmine oil to business meetings. Cleopatra was, and still is, one of the lucky few, as jasmine's exorbitant price ($700 to $900 an ounce) marks it as a precious oil. Some would argue that its ability to generate strength and confidence and its luxurious, long-lasting fragrance make it a worthwhile investment. Just a small amount of jasmine in a carrier oil such as jojoba oil will go a long way. Perfumes with jasmine have always been desirable, so don't deny yourself.

Recommended use: A bath with jasmine is a luxurious way to beat feelings of depression. Rose, sandalwood, and ylang-ylang, among others, can be combined in a bath blend with jasmine, too.

Blends well with: sandalwood, rose, neroli, cypress, juniper, ylang-ylang, and orange.

Caution: Do not take jasmine oil internally. Do not use during the first several months of pregnancy.

Juniper or Juniper Berry *(Juniperus communis)*

Juniper essential oil is extracted by steam-distillation of the ripe berries of the juniper bush, which can be found in Canada and Europe, especially Italy. This essential oil possesses a powerful, fresh, and fruity or pine aroma. Juniper berries are well known as the flavoring of gin, although the essential oil uses the dried berries.

Juniper essential oil has toning and stimulating properties. Juniper has been known since ancient times for its strong antiseptic and diuretic properties. The essential oil is used to detoxify and cleanse the body and is also known to be parasitical (a parasite destroyer). It has, in fact, been used for hundreds of years as a household disinfectant. It is also an astringent oil used in baths and massage oils for treating cellulite. It can be used to treat hemorrhoids and urinary tract infections, and is reputed to boost the immune system. Juniper is said to reduce swelling and relieve the pain of arthritis. It is also believed to restore psychic purity and calm emotions, especially at times when emotions are vulnerable and you are experiencing low energy. Traditionally, juniper was believed to possess magical qualities, and has been used to protect one from evil. Juniper is also wonderful in skin care and hair oil blends.

Recommended use: For a detoxifying bath blend, try five drops of juniper with three drops of grapefruit oil. Add to a warm bath and mix well. Some say regular use of these oils can help get rid of cellulite, too. A vaporizer with a few drops of juniper can help a sick child suffering from croup or whooping cough.

Blends well with: rosemary, grapefruit, eucalyptus, lavender, and jasmine.

Caution: Avoid during pregnancy. Avoid if you suffer from kidney problems.

Labdanum

See **Rockrose.**

Lavandin *(Lavandula x intermedia)*

This is an essential oil of a hybrid of true lavender and spike lavender which is extracted by steam-distillation from the flowering tops. These aromatic plants produce an oil that is very similar to other lavenders, but with a more camphorlike scent.

Lavandin also acts much the same as lavender, being a particularly good oil for a multitude of ailments, including the treatment of headaches, muscle pain, colds, and sinus problems. It can be used in baths, massage oils, and in inhalations. Lavandin is not as powerful an oil as lavender; it also does not have lavender's strong sedating effect, making it a good daytime oil.

Recommended uses: Use in a warm bath to soothe achy muscles or inhale to relieve headache pain.

Blends well with: geranium, clary sage, thyme, patchouli, marjoram, rosemary, and most citrus oils, especially lime and bergamot.

*Lavender *(Lavender officinalis* or *Lavandula augustifolia)*, True Lavender *(Lavendula vera)*, or Spike Lavender *(Lavandula spica)*

Considered the most indispensible and versatile essential oil, lavender essential oil is extracted by steam-distillation from the flowering tops of many different types of lavender, producing varying quality and aromas. The plants can be found in France, Italy, and England. Lavender grows best in high altitudes; in fact, the higher the altitude, the finer the quality of the essential oil. True lavender traditionally comes from England. French lavender, a smaller plant not found in cold climates, also produces a wonderful oil. Spike lavender is not as strong, but it produces three times as much oil and has a more prominent, camphorlike aroma.

Lavender's familiar sweet, clean, fresh scent is a telling description, as the word lavender has its origins in the Latin *lavare,* to wash. It is well documented that lavender was employed to perfume the baths and underwear of the Romans and was used for at least 1,000 years in various folk remedies.

Often referred to as *blue magic,* lavender has a regenerative effect on the nervous system, bringing about feelings of calm and aiding sleeplessness. It is a most valued oil for its beneficial effect on insomnia and relieving tension or migraine headaches. Lavender is wonderful when used to scent the air, linens, or in a warm, luxurious bath where it will aid the release of muscle tension and help you get to sleep.

Truly multitalented, lavender oil is frequently used to relieve emotional stress, anxiety, nervous conditions, tension, or mental fatigue. Its gentle floral aroma can help balance mood swings, panic, and depression. It can be a workaholic's best friend and can be very beneficial to people who find themselves being overly analytical as it helps allay feelings of worry, fear, and impatience.

It is particularly helpful in the treatment of burns or scalds (remember Gattefosse's experiment?), promoting healing and preventing scarring, and it is also a powerful remedy for cuts, wounds, and bites. Lavender oil is a natural antiseptic, antibiotic, antiviral, bactericide, antispasmodic, antidepressant, and it has a lightly sedating effect.

According to recent tests at the Smell and Taste Treatment and Research Foundation in Chicago, the scent of lavender seems to increase the brain's alpha wave function, which resembles the type of activity associated with a relaxed state. Lavender oil is considered a pioneer oil because of its healing properties. It promotes new cell growth and relieves headaches. Some say it can lower high blood pressure. Lavender is a great oil to have on hand during childbirth. It can even be used in a massage oil to help prevent stretch marks.

Lavender is an oil known to increase activity of the other oils with which it is blended, and it blends well with almost any other essential oil. Folklore has it that the aroma of lavender can help to calm untamed lions and tigers. (Imagine what it can do for your spouse!) In ancient times, lavender was believed to ensure fidelity. According to another study conducted by the Smell and Taste Treatment and Research Foundation, the combined aromas of pumpkin pie and lavender are a sexual turn-on. The men in the study group were monitored for penile blood flow while wearing odorized masks. The study showed that their blood flow increased rather dramatically whenever the combined scents of pumpkin pie and lavender were released. No matter what your reason, even if you try no other essential oil, no home should be without lavender.

Lavender is a very gentle oil and is recognized as one of the only essential oils that is safe to use undiluted (neat) on the skin. (Note: People with skin sensitivities and allergies should always use caution when applying any essential oil. Do a patch test to be safe.)

Recommended uses: Bath: Use three to five drops in a warm bath and soak for twenty minutes to calm and relax.

Neat application: Place a drop on each temple to relieve a headache or directly to a bee sting to relieve the pain and to help you calm down.

Diffuser: Put three to five drops in a diffuser pot to calm and relax you and to scent your room.

Inhalation: Inhale the scent of lavender directly from the bottle or place two or three drops on a tissue and carry it with you. At the first sign of stress or a panic attack, inhale deeply. For restful sleep, add a drop or two to the outer corner of your pillow at bedtime. To help kids ease into a pleasant slumber, put a drop or two on their pajamas before bedtime.

Fresh-smelling laundry: Place a few drops of lavender oil on a damp washcloth and throw it into the clothes dryer with your laundry. Your linens and clothes will smell fresh and clean.

Blends well with: almost all other oils, especially citrus and other floral scents.

Lemon *(Citrus limonum)*

Lemon essential oil is cold-pressed from the outer rind of the fruit, which comes mainly from the Mediterranean, especially Southern Italy, as well as America. Depending on the time of harvest, it can take as many as 3,000 lemons to produce just two pounds of the essential oil, so needles to say, this oil is rather expensive. The hand-pressed oil is usually of a finer quality than machine-pressed oil. Hand-pressing, in fact, is a game the whole family can play. The women and children are charged with cutting the fruit and scraping out the flesh. The men take care of the pressing.

This rejuvenating oil is an astringent and antiseptic that is good for itchy skin conditions, such as eczema, or for oily skin. Add lemon oil drops to a sponge bath for problem skin. Lemon essential oil cleanses, refreshes, cools, and stimulates. It can be used to condition nails and cuticles and can also lighten stained hands. It eases stress, anxiety, tension, or mental fatigue and is considered an energizing, uplifting aroma that activates the body. In a recent Japanese experiment, a company piped a lemon scent into their offices via the building ventilators. They noted a 53 percent decline in clerical errors. Lemon essential oil is very rich in vitamin C and vitamin A (in the form of carotene). Lemon is a tonic to the lymphatic and digestive systems. It is believed to help break up cellulite when used in massage. Lemon is a detoxifying agent that can be used in a diffuser to purify your home (think of all the household cleaners on the market that have a lemon, albeit synthetic, scent added).

Lemon essential oil mixes well with geranium and immortelle to curb your desire for cigarettes and to detoxify your system from the adverse effects that smoking has caused. Lemon oil is great in a room spray or in a bath.

Recommended uses: Add five or six drops of lemon essential oil to sudsy water when doing dishes by hand. It will not only cut the grease from the dishes, but will also smell great. Add a few drops of lemon oil to a spray bottle filled with water. Spray the room for a fresh-smelling environment. Also try a blend of lemon, tea tree, and lavender (ten to twenty drops total). For a refreshing morning bath, combine three drops of lemon essential oil with three drops of rosemary and two drops of eucalyptus. Add to a tub of warm water and mix well.

Blends well with: most other essential oils, especially ylang-ylang and other citrus oils; it also blends well with other fresh scents, including lavender, pine, cedar, eucalyptus, fennel, and juniper.

Caution: Do not use lemon essential oil on the skin in direct sunlight. Dilute to 1 percent and use only three drops in a bath to avoid skin irritation.

Lemon Balm

See **Melissa.**

Lemon Verbena

See **Verbena.**

Lemongrass *(Cymbopogon citratus)*

Lemongrass oil is steam-distilled from the fresh or partly dried leaves of the plant, probably a native of Ceylon and parts of East India. It is cultivated not only in India but also in such areas as Africa, Central America, the West Indies, and South America. This oil possesses a sweet and powerful fresh-grassy, lemony fragrance, making it great for deodorizing a room. It is also a refreshing and cleansing tonic for the body, especially when recovering from an illness. Use lemongrass essential oil to stimulate circulation, deodorize feet, to treat oily skin, and to energize emotionally. It can be used to help with digestive ailments and to reduce flatulence. Used in an aroma lamp or diffuser, lemongrass could be helpful for children who may be prone to rickets. It also makes a potent insect repellent when diffused in a room or as an air spray.

Recommended use: A few drops (see caution below) of lemongrass oil in a warm bath can ease away the tensions of the day, refresh and rejuvenate, even through jet lag or PMS.

Blends well with: pine, eucalyptus, juniper, geranium, lavender, and lime.

Caution: Lemongrass can cause skin irritation, so test first on sensitive skin. Dilute to 1 percent and use only three drops in a bath.

Lime *(Citrus aurantifolia)*

Lime essential oil is extracted by steam-distillation of the chopped fruit or the skin of the lime. It has a fresh, lively, tangy aroma that is similar to, yet different from lemon. This refreshing essential oil is considered a tonic to the immune system, cools fever, stimulates appetite, and heightens mental clarity. It is also an excellent astringent for greasy skin, helps control bleeding, and is a natural deodorant. It is a cheering oil, one that is refreshing to tired bodies and uplifting for depression. When blended with such oils as ylang-ylang, vanilla, or tonka bean, lime essential oil takes on a sensual feel. This oil acts in a similar way to lemon and other citrus oils.

Recommended use: To deodorize your kitchen, add one drop of lime essential oil to a washing cloth when you are cleaning kitchen surfaces.

Blends well with: ylang-ylang, vanilla, tonka bean, and other citrus oils.

Caution: Test first on sensitive skin. Lime can cause spots on the skin if exposed to sunlight.

Mandarin *(Citrus nobilis)*

The essential oil of mandarin is produced by cold-pressing the outer skin. Its aroma is delicate and very similar to that of the fruit itself, which supposedly got its name because it was once a traditional gift offered to the Chinese mandarins.

Gentle and calming, this mild essential oil is good for relieving insomnia and nervous tension. It is also used in the care of oily skin and can be used in massage for the digestive system, as well as to help prevent stretch marks. It is known in France as the children's remedy because of its mildness. This oil can be used safely during pregnancy.

Recommended use: To aid with convalescence, try mandarin oil in a room diffuser. It should help calm nerves. Mandarin can be used in a bath or footbath blend for kids. Try a footbath blend of two drops each of mandarin, vanilla, and ylang-ylang.

Blends well with: other citrus oils.

Caution: Do not use on the skin in direct sunlight.

Marjoram or Sweet Marjoram *(Origanum marjorana)*

Essential oil of marjoram is extracted by steam-distillation of the leaves and flowering tops of this small, hardy plant, and it is mainly exported from France. Sweet marjoram was used medicinally by ancient Greek physicians, and in fragrances and cosmetics.

This essential oil is used to treat stress, anxiety, tension, mental fatigue, and migraine headaches. It is a very strong sedative and an anaphrodisiac (that is, it turns off sexual desire, perhaps because if you smell too much of it, you'll fall right off to sleep). It is a warm, soothing, uplifting scent, and has commonly been used as a comforting remedy for grief, confusion, and melancholy. Marjoram is believed to feed one's need for nurturance and affection.

It is useful on tired muscles and rheumatic pain, especially when added to an aftersports rub; it is also useful for massaging on the abdomen during menstruation. It is very relaxing when used in a hot bath, especially blended with lavender, bergamot, and rosewood. Traditionally, marjoram has been believed to bring longevity. Mythology has it that the goddess Venus gave marjoram its magical fragrance.

Recommended use: Put a drop or two on a tissue and inhale it when you need comforting or add a couple of drops to the outside edges of your pillow before bedtime to help you fall asleep. (Drops should be placed so that the oil does not come in direct contact with the skin.)

Mixes well with: lavender, bergamot, chamomile, cypress, cedarwood, rosemary, and tea tree.

Caution: Marjoram should not be used by pregnant women. It is a strong sedative, so caution should be taken. Use sparingly.

Melissa or Lemon Balm *(Melissa officinalis)*

Used since antiquity in the Middle East, this expensive, lemon-scented essential oil is extracted from all parts of *Melissa officinalis,* a popular garden herb, which for centuries has been associated with the treatment of anxiety, tension, asthma, coughs, circulation problems, and heart ailments. It is most often used in an aroma lamp or other diffuser. Experts recommend that you buy this oil through an aromatherapist or other reputable source, or you may get an oil produced from a plant such as lemongrass.

Melissa is an antispasmodic and a nerve sedative. While it is calming and soothing, it also has an uplifting effect on the mind and body. Smelling the essential oil of melissa produces a calming influence on the brain's limbic system, which controls the nervous system and protects the brain from becoming overstimulated. This is a great oil to use during the winter cold season, as well as during pollen season. Melissa, in fact, is highly recommended as a treatment of allergies, especially whenever chamomile has not worked. It is often used in preparations for skin infections, and it can also be effective in room sprays and insect repellents.

Recommended use: For a relaxing massage oil, combine two drops of melissa with ten drops of lavender and seven drops of clary sage. Add to two ounces of carrier oil.

Mixes well with: lavender, geranium, and other floral oils, and with most citrus oils.

Caution: Never take melissa internally. Do not use it on the skin in direct sunlight. This oil contains citronellol, which can cause skin irritation in some people. Dilute it to 1 percent and use only three drops in a bath to avoid skin irritation.

Mimosa *(Acacia dealbata)*

The solvent extraction of mimosa produces a concrete and an absolute, which come from the flowers and twigs of this plant. Both the concrete and the absolute are mainly produced in Italy and the south of France. This woody-floral fragrance is used in many top-of-the-line perfumes.

Mimosa is antiseptic and astringent, making it effective in skin care treatments, especially for oily and sensitive skin types. It is also useful in keeping anxiety, stress, and nervous tension in check.

Recommended use: Add several drops to a body oil blend to moisturize skin.

Blends well with: benzoin, lavandin, lavender, ylang-ylang, violet, and most floral and spice oils.

Myrrh *(Commiphora myrrha)*

Myrrh is a sap or resin rather than a true essential oil, which comes from the myrrh tree. Originally from northeast Africa and Arabia, Egyptians burned this smoky, mysterious oil as incense every day in religious ceremonies and sun-worshipping rituals and used it in medicinal preparations, as well as in creams, ointments, and for embalming practices. Like frankincense, myrrh is one of the herbs mentioned in the Bible (it was in the Garden of Eden) and was an ancient trading commodity that figured prominently in personal perfumes and religious rituals. It is believed to be rejuvenating and uplifting. Legend says it promotes faithfulness.

Many aromatherapists say that it is excellent for oral hygiene, mouth ulcers, and gingivitis when added to gargle or mouthwash. It's an antiseptic, astringent, tonic, and a healing agent that can be used to treat coughs, digestive troubles, infections, wounds, skin fungus, and cracked skin or eczema.

Recommended uses: Add to a cream for protecting your skin against chapping in the cold. To treat cuts, apply a solution of five drops of myrrh essential oil and two teaspoons of cooled, boiled water.

Blends well with: frankincense, sandalwood, peppermint, lavender, thyme, pine, benzoin, cypress, juniper, mandarin, and spice oils.

Caution: Do not use myrrh during pregnancy.

Myrtle *(Myrtus communis)*

This essential oil, which comes mainly from the Mediterranean region, is extracted by steam-distillation of the leaves and twigs and sometimes the flowering tips of branches. It has a sweet herby scent that is somewhat reminiscent of eucalyptus. Myrtle can be used to treat acne, hemorrhoids, and oily skin, as well as respiratory conditions such as asthma, bronchitis, and chronic coughs. Myrtle is sometimes used to strengthen the immune system, so it is a good choice for treating colds, flu, and other infectious diseases. It is a mild oil that also has a slight sedative effect so it can help one relax.

Recommended use: Use in a diffuser at night to combat coughs and other respiratory conditions—for adults and children alike.

Blends well with: pine, lavender, lemon, neroli, and cypress.

*Neroli or Orange Blossom *(Citrus aurantium)*

Neroli or orange blossom essential oil is extracted by steam-distillation or sometimes enfleurage from fresh orange flowers of the bitter orange tree. It has a rich, bittersweet, yet somewhat spicy fragrance. It is named after Anna Maria de la Trémoille, the seventeenth-century Italian Princess of Nerola, who used it to perfume her gloves, lace shawls, and baths.

This very relaxing and uplifting essential oil relieves stress, anxiety, depression, tension, and mental fatigue. Gentle neroli is good for calming butterflies in the stomach and is an especially good oil for people who become upset over small matters. It is also recommended for shock or as relief for disorders that are brought on by a sudden fright, which could put a strain on the heart.

According to many sources, neroli is not an aphrodisiac per se, but it does help in the area of sexual relations due to its calming effects. Neroli is useful in relieving the nervous anxiety often felt before a sexual encounter. This can explain the presence of orange blossoms in bridal wreaths of long ago.

Neroli oil can be wonderfully soothing in a warm bath. It is also good for circulation, cell regeneration, and skin elasticity, and it can be used to treat dry sensitive skin, scarring, and stretch marks. This is one of the most expensive oils, but it is still used in many fragrances.

Recommended use: Add five drops to an aroma lamp or diffuser overnight for a good night's sleep and for a psychological pick-me-up.

Blends well with: sandalwood, cedar, lavender, lemon, and with other floral oils, such as jasmine, rose, and geranium.

Niaouli *(Melalenca viridiflora)*

The essential oil of niaouli is extracted by steam-distillation of the leaves of the niaouli tree. Niaouli is the modern name for gomenol, named after Gomen in New Caledonia, where the oil originates. It has a sweet, fresh aroma, somewhat similar to eucalyptus. It can be used for treating cuts and wounds, burns, infections, skin irritations, and acne, if used with a carrier oil or in a skin tonic. It has long been considered an effective medicine for treating boils. In fact, at one time it was issued to legionnaires in the French Foreign Legion. It is also good as a chest rub and, when vaporized, to treat sinusitis, as well as colds, flu, sore throats, bronchitis, and other respiratory problems.

The oil is a strong antiseptic not only for the bronchial system but for the urinary tract, and it even serves as a good room disinfectant.

Recommended use: As a wash for cleaning minor wounds, add five drops of niaouli oil to one half pint boiled and cooled water. Wash the area as often as necessary.

Blends well with: hyssop, pine, lemon, myrtle, orange, and eucalyptus.

Note: Many experts say that true oil of niaouli may be used safely neat (undiluted) on the skin. Beware, however, of some adulterated forms on the market, which have other elements added to them.

Nutmeg and Mace *(Myristica fragrans)*

The spicy aroma of the essential oil of nutmeg can best be described as nutmeglike. It is extracted by steam- or water-distillation of the dried, ground-up seeds (for nutmeg) and dried seed coverings (for mace). The tree is an evergreen that is native to the Moluccas. Used to treat stress, anxiety, tension, or mental fatigue, it calms the body and is therefore good for insomnia. (Think of the spice sprinked on hot chocolate before bedtime.) It is believed to be good for the intestinal tract and reproductive organs. Some say it can even reverse male impotency and hair loss.

Recommended use: Use in a diffuser to scent the air, either on its own or in combination with a citrus aroma such as orange.

Blends well with: orange, mandarin, coriander, lavandin, geranium, clary sage, rosemary, lime, and petitgrain.

Caution: Avoid nutmeg and mace oils during pregnancy. Also, large quantities have been shown to be toxic, causing hallucinations. Do not inhale these oils for long periods of time, and do not use them in a bath. The oils can be dangerous if taken internally. Nutmeg and mace oils are best left to the experts; consult a licensed aromatherapist before using them.

Orange, Sweet *(Citrus sinensis)*

The essential oil of orange has the familiar sweet, citrusy fragrance of the fruit, and is extracted by cold-pressing the fruit's skin. At one time, orange trees were rather rare and were native to China and India. Today, the oil is produced mainly in Israel, Cyprus, Brazil, and North America. An antidepressant, orange is sometimes referred to as a cheering oil, especially pleasant during the wintertime. Children love sweet orange. It is a sedative, calms the stomach, helps diarrhea and constipation, lowers cholesterol and it lifts your spirits and turns depression into joy. It is an excellent skin tonic and is believed to brighten a dull complexion. It is good for sore muscles and insomnia. Blend sweet orange with spicy essential oils for a soothing, uplifting bath. Add it to a massage oil to help the digestive system. In high doses, this aroma might produce a feeling of sleepiness. Like all citrus oils, orange oil has a short life. Store it in a cool, dry place, such as the refrigerator. Sweet orange essential oil is relatively inexpensive, so you can even use it for cleaning the house.

Recommended uses: Mix a few drops with water in a spray bottle and spritz to deodorize a room, as well as to combat melancholy. Combine two drops of sweet orange with two drops of vanilla. Add to a warm bath for a child. Mix well. (It smells like a creamsicle!) For grown-ups, add a few drops of frankincense to this mix.

Blends well with: cinnamon, clove, clary sage, lavender, lemon, neroli, and myrrh.

Caution: Some sweet orange oil is distilled from the outer peel. Although the distilled orange essential oil is phototoxic and should not be used on skin in direct sunlight, the expressed sweet orange essential oil is not known to be phototoxic.

Palmarosa *(Cymbopogon martini)*

A light, uplifting floral aroma, palmarosa essential oil is steam-distilled or water-distilled from a wild-growing scented grass that is related to lemongrass and citronella. A native to India and Pakistan, this herbaceous plant is also grown in Brazil and Central America. With its refreshing scent that can be described as something between rose and geranium, it is said to bring clarity of mind and is known as a great skin care oil when mixed with a sweet almond carrier oil. It is believed to regenerate the cellular body. It moisturizes, so it is especially beneficial to mature skin and for acne and eczema.

Palmarosa has been used to regulate the thyroid and to treat anorexia. It is considered a tonic for the entire system. It is an exotic yet inexpensive oil that is sometimes used to adulterate rose oil, which is extremely costly. Like rose, palmarosa is believed to attract love.

Recommended use: For mature skin, add palmarosa essential oil to a body oil blend made with sweet almond oil (twenty drops of essential oil to two ounces of carrier oil).

Blends well with: geranium, rosewood, sandalwood, cedarwood, and most floral oils.

Parsley *(Petroselinum sativum)*

Essential oil of parsley is extracted through steam-distillation of the whole plant and also its seeds. Parsley, best known as a common herb used in cooking, produces an oil with a spicy-herby scent that is very similar to the familiar plant. This oil is produced primarily in Europe, especially France, Germany, Hungary, and The Netherlands.

Its main uses in aromatherapy are in the treatments of ailments falling within the circulatory, digestive, and genitourinary systems. Among its many actions, parsley is antirheumatic, antiseptic, astringent, carminative, diuretic, and a mild stimulant. Parsley oil can be helpful in treating arthritis, rheumatism, indigestion, and to fight cystitis and urinary tract infections.

For skin care, parsley essential oil can be toning, stimulating, and cleansing. It is especially beneficial for oily skin and skin with impurities. It is also useful in cellulite treatments. Parsley oil is also vasoconstricting, meaning it helps promote the contraction of broken blood vessels.

Recommended use: Add parsley oil to a skin oil or cream to help contract broken blood vessels. (Note: This treatment would have to continue over a sustained period of time.)

Blends well with: clary sage, rose, orange blossom, tea tree, and most spice oils.

Caution: Use parsley essential oil in moderation, as it can be somewhat toxic and irritating. Avoid during pregnancy.

Patchouli *(Pogostemon patchouli)*

Patchouli essential oil is extracted by steam distillation of the dried leaves of this small Indian plant. If you were a hippy in the free love '60s, you might recognize the smell of this earthy, musky exotic (some say strange or offbeat) oil, since adulterated versions of this aroma were used to cover the smell of marijuana smoke. Others recognize this scent from their grandmother's closet, and many describe the aroma as being a musty attic smell. Patchouli has been used for centuries in China, India, and Malaysia for medicinal purposes. East Indians have long used patchouli to add fragrance to textiles. This is an aroma you either love or hate.

It is said that the scent of patchouli is a repellent against moths. During the Victorian era, in fact, linens and cashmere shawls exported from India to Britain were packed in boxes containing patchouli leaves. It is still used in the East to scent linens and clothes. It is an antidepressant and tissue regenerator. Pure patchouli oil is believed to soothe and uplift the spirit and to be a grounding aroma when we find ourselves under stress and emotions run out of control. Patchouli is a sedative oil if used in small amounts, and stimulating if higher dosages are used. Patchouli's aroma is known to help clarify objectives and break through confusion. It is an oil that some say will fight off feelings of apathy and will be reassuring if you feel neglected.

It is useful in protecting and moisturizing dry, mature, or blemished skin. Earthy and sensuous, patchouli is also supposed to be an aphrodisiac (but only if both partners like the smell). Patchouli oil can also be used on the scalp to help control dandruff.

Recommended uses: For a facial oil for inflamed skin, add fifteen drops of patchouli, five drops of myrrh, and one drop of clove to two ounces of carrier oil (jojoba with 10 percent wheat germ oil and vitamin E). For mature skin, try ten drops each of patchouli and frankincense with the carrier blend.

Blends well with: lemon, ylang-ylang, frankincense, jasmine, and rose.

*Peppermint *(Mentha piperta)*

Peppermint essential oil is produced by steam-distillation of the leaves and flowering tops of a small plant that is grown in temperate climates, including the United States. The quality can vary greatly depending on soil conditions and climate. Peppermint, which contains menthol, was used by ancient Egyptians and Israelites for its cooling effect.

Herbalists in ancient Egypt, Greece, and Rome were known to have used peppermint for a wide variety of medical ailments.

Peppermint oil is one of the most important essential oils, especially for digestive problems. Even Hippocrates, the father of medicine, advocated peppermint for its stimulant and diuretic properties. Peppermint is a general tonic that stimulates, refreshes, cools, restores, and uplifts the mind and the body. Peppermint's invigorating aroma is an excellent antidote to overwork and mental fatigue. It can really help clear your head. It is used to treat stress, anxiety, depression, and tension. It is also antispasmodic and analgesic, relieving pain, indigestion, flatulence, nausea, asthma, bronchial spasms, and tension headaches. It's great for refreshing tired feet, helps treat the common cold and fainting, and can aid with concentration. It is also useful for treating inflammation. One of its best-known uses is that it is said to cheer up children.

Inhale this essence to clear your sinuses, or add it to a massage blend to aid the digestive system. Some experts say to add a few drops to the car dashboard to help stay alert and fresh while driving. The heat of the car will help diffuse the scent.

Recommended uses: Take a quick sniff right from the bottle to become more alert on a long trip. Peppermint oil is great in a morning bath blend with rosemary and juniper or on its own in a cool bath (use only two or three drops).

Blends well with: lavender and eucalyptus.

Caution: Avoid during pregnancy, especially during the first three months. Experts say not to use more than three drops in a bath to avoid skin irritation. Peppermint (like eucalyptus) is contraindicated with homeopathic medicines, so use either the essential oil or the homeopathic remedy. Do not store essential oils near homeopathic medicine.

Petitgrain *(Citrus aurantium)*

This lovely, fresh-scented oil is from the same tree as neroli/orange blossom and has similar properties, but petitgrain is steam-distilled from the leaves or twigs instead of the petals. It restores, relaxes, cleanses, and uplifts the spirit and helps to relieve anxiety, stress, and insomnia. It also has insecticidal, deodorant, antiseptic, and tonic properties. Inhale the undiluted oil to stimulate the mind and help with memory. Two drops are great in a final rinse for healthy hair. It is very useful in treating sunburn and itchy skin. It is less expensive to produce than neroli, so it is often used as a substitute.

Recommended use: For a refreshing bath, add several drops of petitgrain essential oil to warm water. It can be used on its own or blended with rosemary. This combination can also be used successfully in a hair rinse.

Blends well with: bergamot, rosemary, geranium, lavender, sweet orange, and neroli.

Caution: Petitgrain essential oil may cause skin discoloration if used on skin and exposed to sunlight.

Pine *(Pinus sylvestris)*

The essential oil of pine comes from the needles, young twigs, and cones of the Scotch or Norwegian pine tree, which grows most readily in northern regions of the world, especially Finland. There are several other species of pine, but this is the one most closely associated with aromatherapy treatments. This oil has a strong, fresh aroma that has a powerful antiseptic quality. In fact, it is sometimes used in a vaporizer in hospital burn units and has been shown to combat infection after serious burns. It can be used to treat stress, anxiety, tension, or mental fatigue. A powerful expectorant, it is particularly valuable in treating coughs, colds, sore throats, bronchitis, and just about any respiratory problems. For home use, its best application methods are diffusers and steam inhalations, especially for treating chest infections.

For healing purposes, it can be mixed very successfully with tea tree or eucalyptus, or it can be used on its own. Pine oil is also believed to help relieve rheumatic pain, as it is a stimulating oil for the circulatory system. Pine is a powerful cleanser, not just for the mind and body, but for your environment as well. As anyone who has ever used a commercial housecleaning product knows, pine is an excellent deodorant and purifying agent.

Recommended use: Add about ten drops of pine essential oil to your bucket of warm, sudsy water, and go about your housecleaning. Once you've tried the pure oil, you'll never want to go back to synthetics again.

Blends well with: cinnamon, eucalyptus, and tea tree.

Caution: Always dilute pine to avoid skin irritation. People with very sensitive skin, including sufferers of eczema and dermatitis, should avoid contact with this oil.

Rockrose or Labdanum *(Cistus ladaniferus)*

Rockrose essential oil is derived by steam-distillation of the gum, the absolute, or from the plant's leaves and twigs. Labdanum is a resin that is extracted by solvent extraction. The oil, with a sweet, herbaceous scent, is produced mainly in Spain. It was used as an ingredient in beauty creams in ancient Egypt, and has been used since the Middle Ages for medicinal purposes.

Rockrose (or labdanum) is used mainly for perfumery, and in fact it is a fixative for perfumes. It is a strong oil with antiseptic, astringent, and tonic properties. It is especially good for mature skin, acne, and oily skin, as well as for abdominal disorders and respiratory ailments such as colds, coughs, and bronchitis.

Recommended use: A sitz bath with rockrose and marjoram (equal parts) can be useful in treating such abdominal problems as cystitis or menstrual cramps.

Blends well with: clary sage, pine, juniper, lavender, bergamot, sandalwood, patchouli, and cypress.

Caution: Avoid during pregnancy.

*Rose *(Rosa damascena, Rosa centifolia, and Rosa gallica)*

> You may break, you may shatter the vase, if you will,
> But the scent of the roses will hang round still.
> Thomas Moore, *Farewell! But Whenever*

The rose, the queen of the flowers, produces an essential oil that truly stands apart from the rest. Smell a rose and you will instantly feel uplifted (unless, of course, you associate the smell of roses with some unpleasant incident). The essential oil is extracted by steam-distillation of fresh flowers. To produce just one pound of the essential oil takes about 5,000 pounds of flowers, so needless to say, rose oil is one of the most expensive oils. There are many different types of roses from all around the globe. The most expensive rose essence is rose otto, which is produced in Bulgaria. Another popular rose essence, rose de mai, comes from Grasse in southern France.

Rose is emotionally soothing, so it is widely used to treat stress, depression, anxiety, tension, anger, mental fatigue, and sexual tensions. It helps maintain self-confidence and encourages feelings of self-love. It is an excellent skin regenerator (tones and cleanses) and is often used in skin care treatments, especially beneficial for dry or mature skin or inflamed skin. Other uses include treatment for nausea, headaches, and insomnia. Among its therapeutic properties are antibacterial, antidepressant, astringent, sedative, and a tonic for the heart, stomach, liver, and uterus. Rose is very good for all hormonal imbalances in women, and it is excellent in a bath or masage oil for treating many gynecological problems, including those relating to PMS, menopause, and infertility. Rose is most famous, however (thanks to Cleopatra) as an aphrodisiac. She would fill her room knee-deep with rose petals, awaiting Mark Antony.

Used by the Romans and Egyptians, it has been known throughout the ages to possess very sensual and healing elements. Bouquets of roses have been discovered in the tomb of Tutankhamen. The discovery of rose otto can be traced to the 1590s, when a canal was dug for the wedding of a Persian princess, or so the story goes. The waters of the canal were strewn with tons of rose petals. When the bridal couple went rowing out on the aromatic water, they found an oily substance with a lovely sweet fragrance floating on top. This led to the collection and then production of otto of rose and the Persians apparently were leaders in this field for hundreds of years.

To enjoy the rose essential oil, inhale it directly from the bottle to alleviate feelings of anger or stress. Also try a couple of drops on a handkerchief and inhale the aroma. To make this very expensive oil go a long way, however, use a candle diffuser. You only need a small amount of the exquisite oil to achieve great effects. Rose essential oil can be very sticky at room temperature and it goes solid at relatively high temperatures. Using the rose flower water (rosewater) is another alternative. Rosewater is a by-product of the steam-distillation process used to obtain rose essential oil. The water is saturated with many of the beneficial properties of the rose. It is particularly useful in rejuvenating skin, and it is very soothing.

Pure rose essential oil is seldom used in commercial products since it is so expensive. Instead, a cheaper synthetic is used. Many people are actually surprised when they smell the real rose oil for the first time. But make no mistake, a rose by any other name does not smell the same—or act the same. Don't be fooled by cheap imitations; there is no substitute for the real thing.

Recommended uses: To relieve symptoms of PMS, add six or seven drops of rose oil to one half ounce of carrier oil and use it in a warm bath. Soak for ten minutes. Or, use this blend to rub onto your stomach or back. For a relaxing, luxurious bath, use two drops of rose oil combined with five drops of lavender and two drops of ylang-ylang. For normal skin, try a facial oil made with ten drops of rose oil and five drops each of geranium and rosewood. Blend into two ounces of carrier oil, such as jojoba with 10 percent wheat germ and vitamin E.

Blends well with: neroli, lavender, sandalwood, and jasmine.
Caution: Avoid during the first four months of pregnancy.

*Rosemary *(Rosemarinus officinalis)*

The essential oil from rosemary has a camphorlike aroma and is extracted by steam-distillation of the flowers and leaves. This herb is grown in Italy, Spain, the south of France, and North Africa, as well as in America. The ancient Egyptians and many people since have found that rosemary essential oil is a true pick-me-up.

This popular aromatherapy oil can be used to treat stress, anxiety, tension, or mental fatigue. Rosemary is a physical and mental stimulant, known to revive, warm, and restore. It is great for writer's block or for students studying for exams, as it helps with memory and concentration. Throughout history, rosemary has been known as the herb for remembrance. In Ancient Greece and Rome, students would adorn their heads with wreaths of rosemary when engaging in their studies. (I recommend using the essential oil in a diffuser instead.) The Greeks and Romans believed rosemary to be a sacred plant that possessed magical powers.

Invigorating and refreshing, rosemary is very useful in treating a wide variety of ailments, including muscular aches and pains, poor circulation, arthritis, rheumatism, depression, boredom, disorientation, fatigue, memory loss, migraine, headaches, coughs, colds, flu, rheumatism, gout, skin problems, constipation, and diabetes. Rosemary is also known as a stimulant (both general and of the hormones produced by the adrenal glands), a lung antiseptic, a decongestant, and even an insect repellent. It works well in a diffuser to clear a stuffy room. Rosemary is said to improve all the senses, and it is an oil that reportedly helps build self-confidence and allows us to set ourselves on a clear path.

Used through the ages as an important ingredient in beauty and health preparations, rosemary has been turning up in many contemporary beauty treatments such as hair care products and acne and cellulite remedies. Rosemary will bring out color highlights in dark hair and it is thought to be a great hair tonic as it improves circulation to the scalp. It could also help control dandruff problems and restore suppleness and shine to the hair. Try using it in a carrier oil for a scalp massage. It is known as the dew of the sea with good reason. Rosemary loves to grow near the sea. *Ros* means dew, and *marinums* means of the sea.

The queen of Hungary is supposed to have used a distilled essence of rosemary in her daily bath. She was reportedly so beautiful at age seventy-two that she enchanted the king of Poland, who promptly asked her to be his bride. This perfume water, called Hungary water, is the oldest known, and versions of it are still being made today.

Recommended uses: Place one or two drops on a cotton ball and inhale the aroma while studying. To refresh your memory, sniff again for recall. Rosemary also works well if combined with geranium, an antidepressant. Mix rosemary oil in a diffuser pot with a few drops of sweet orange to clean and refresh the air.

Blends well with: peppermint, sweet orange, basil, pine, lemon, juniper, geranium, cedarwood, and bergamot.

Caution: Avoid rosemary during pregnancy, especially during the first three months. Do not use it if you suffer from high blood pressure or epilepsy. Rosemary oil can also cause skin irritation.

Rosewood *(Aniba roseaodora)*

Rosewood essential oil, with its sweet, flowery (some say woodsy) aroma, is relaxing and deodorizing. It is produced by steam-distillation of wood chips from a tree that grows in the rain forests of Brazil. An uplifting antidepressant, it is beneficial to the nervous system and is sometimes used to remedy tiredness, nervousness, and stress. A good antiseptic, it is effective for treating dry skin, acne, and is known for its balancing effects. For some, it helps with migraine and other headaches and with relieving sore muscles. Rosewood is sometimes used to fight off the beginning phases of colds and flu. It is especially useful for students during exam time. Rosewood is a good oil to use as a carpet freshener. Once called bois de rose, these days it is infrequently referred to by that name.

Unfortunately, the rosewood tree supply is quickly being diminished, causing the oil to become harder to come by. Some aromatherapy experts believe that the environmentally correct thing to do is not to use rosewood oil for a while, until the supply can be replenished.

Recommended use: Add a couple of drops of rosewood essential oil to your hairbrush and run it through your hair for a great aroma all day.

Blends well with: bergamot, palmarosa, sandalwood, frankincense, and clary sage, especially for a bath blend.

Sage *(Salvia officinalis)*

This essential oil is distilled from the sun-dried leaves of this seemingly ubiquitous herb. There are about five hundred different varieties of sage, which is grown just about everywhere. The Romans labeled sage *herba sacra,* which means sacred herb, a testament to its powerful healing properties.

Those properties include tonic, antiseptic, astringent, and

diuretic. It can be used to treat sinus headaches, colds, bronchitis, asthma, bacterial infections, rheumatism, arthritis, sprains, and aching muscles. Sage can also be used to treat such ailments as nervousness and low blood pressure, as well as to heal skin eruptions. Sage oil is believed to have a regulating effect on the central nervous system and is helpful in relieving depression, anxiety, and exhaustion. It is frequently used to deal with problems resulting from menopause, as sage contains an estrogen or a natural plant hormone. Native American women traditionally have used this herb to help regulate menstruation and to help with digestive disorders. Most aromatherapy treatments turn to the minty clary sage oil as a substitute for sage, as sage oil can be toxic, even in small doses. Sage is generally less costly than clary sage.

Recommended use: Sage oil can be used in an aroma lamp or diffuser to strengthen emotions, but since sage is considered toxic, it is better to use clary sage for aromatherapy purposes.

Blends well with: lavandin, lavender, rosemary, rosewood, hyssop, and lemon.

Caution: Avoid sage during pregnancy. Never use sage if you suffer from epilepsy or high blood pressure. This oil is best left to professional aromatherapists, if used at all.

*Sandalwood *(Santalum album)*

Used in ancient Egypt, sandalwood oil has an exotic, woody, musky fragrance that creates a sensual atmosphere wherever it goes. This essential oil is extracted by steam-distillation of the crushed wood of the parasitic sandalwood tree, found mostly in Australia, the West Indies, and Asia. The best supposedly comes from India, where the Indian government owns the sandalwood trees so as to preserve them. These trees are used almost exclusively for the extraction of essence. In fact, the sandalwood tree has been a sacred object in India since the fifth century B.C. It is mentioned in the Nirukta, which is the oldest religious writing known. Known as a sensual aroma, to some, the woody tone can be somewhat overpowering.

This relaxing oil is said to be spiritually opening and healing. It is said to bring about serenity and is often used to enhance meditation. It is well-known as an antidepressant with its comforting, elevating, even euphoric powers. It stimulates the immune system and is used to prevent sore throats and to combat bronchitis as well as fatigue.

Sandalwood has antiseptic and tonic properties. It is also good for brittle nails when used with bay and lavender. It is great in a bath with eucalyptus to treat urinary tract infections, is good for treating chest infections and bronchitis, and it aids in sleep.

Sandalwood is moisturizing for dry and mature skin and for damaged hair. Many consider sandalwood to be an aphrodisiac, popular with both men and women, and it is sometimes used to treat impotence. Historical accounts say that Josephine used to cover her walls with the fragrance of sandalwood in order to attract Napoleon. Oriental culture considers sandalwood to be a sacred fragrance. Traditionally, sandalwood has been burnt as an aid to meditation and has often been used in religious ceremonies. The wood of the sandalwood tree is sometimes carved and used as decoration in temples for its fragrance. Sandalwood is an aroma used frequently in modern-day perfumes, and it is often an ingredient in incense. Unfortunately, the sandalwood supply is a bit low these days since the supply of sandalwood trees is rapidly being depleted.

Recommended uses: To aid with sleep, use six or seven drops of sandalwood essential oil in a diffuser. For a facial compress for oily skin, blend one drop each of sandalwood and rose with two drops of geranium. Add the oils to two pints of boiled and cooled water.

Blends well with: most essential oils, especially rose, ylang-ylang, benzoin, jasmine, lemon, geranium, verbena, and frankincense.

Tangerine *(Citrus reticulata)*

Tangerine essential oil has a sweet, fruity fragrance and is produced by cold-pressing the outer skin of the fruit. It was brought to the United States in the 1840s from Europe (it was named tangerine in the United States and was called mandarin in Europe). The tangerine is produced mainly in California, Florida, Texas, and Guinea.

The oil is known as a cheering oil, one that gives inspiration to those who use it. This fresh and lively scent is a favorite among children and pregnant women, although many men love it, too. Spiritually, it is considered an oil of purification and one that awakens joy and dissolves negativity. It can be used to relieve stress and treat tension, restlessness, anxiety, fear, depression, and insomnia. Tangerine oil can be used in a massage oil to relieve muscle cramps and is good for PMS. It also balances dry scalp and dandruff conditions while moisturizing hair and skin. Tangerine is beneficial for purifying oily skin, too. Tangerine is a sedative, tonic, antiseptic, and antispasmodic, and it can be used to assist in lymph drainage. Tangerine is a mild oil that is safe for use with babies and children.

Often, the terms *tangerine* and *mandarin* are used interchangeably, although the two have somewhat different characteristics. Tangerine essential oil, for instance, has less body than mandarin. While mandarin is often used in perfumery, tangerine is not. The tangerine fruit is somewhat larger than the mandarin.

Recommended use: Tangerine essential oil can be added to a massage oil to relieve cramped muscles.

Blends well with: sandalwood, bergamot, tonka bean, coriander, and especially with other citrus oils.

Tarragon *(Artemisia dracunculus)*

Tarragon essential oil is steam-distilled from the leaves of this herb, and is produced mainly in the United States, as well as France, Hungary, and the Netherlands. Its aroma is sweet and spicy-green.

Tarragon oil is antispasmodic, antiseptic, carminative, digestive, and a stimulant. Its main uses in aromatherapy are as an aid to the digestive system and the genitourinary system. Tarragon has been used in the treatment of such ailments as anorexia, hiccups, and nervous indigestion, as well in the treatment of premenstrual tension. The familiar aroma of tarragon is also frequently used as a flavor ingredient in many foods.

Recommended use: Tarragon oil can be used in conjunction with other essential oils in a liniment blend to treat pain resulting from rheumatism.

Blends well with: rockrose (labdanum), lavender, vanilla, pine, and basil.

Caution: This oil can be moderately toxic. Avoid using it during pregnancy.

*Tea Tree or Ti Tree *(Melaleuca alternifolia)*

Tea tree essential oil is distilled from the leaves of this indigenous Australian tree. Tea tree is a powerful antiviral, antibacterial, and antifungal essential oil with a medicinal eucalyptus-like aroma. This detoxifying oil can be used to treat many ailments, including boils, warts, burns, colds, candida, genital herpes, ringworm, flu, sunburn, acne, toothaches, gum disease, pyorrhea, and many types of infections, including sinusitis. It is particularly good in a massage oil before and after operations and for treating ear infections and vaginal infections.

The Aborigines have known about the powerful antiseptic properties of the tea tree, and they have been using it in medications for hundreds of years. Tea tree has seen a resurgence in popularity in modern aromatherapy. It is an immune system enhancer and is cleansing for the skin. A very strong antiseptic, it is great for vaporizing to kill airborne germs. Most agree that it is gentle to the skin* and speeds up healing of external sores, scratches, rashes, and wounds. Tea tree is an excellent oil for treating athlete's foot, foot odor, and dandruff.

Recommended uses: For athlete's foot, be sure to first dry the area thoroughly, then apply four to ten drops of undi-

---

Note: The verdict is still not in regarding applying tea tree directly to the skin. Some say it's O.K., others disagree, stating that tea tree can cause skin sensitization. Consult with a trained aromatherapist if in doubt.

luted tea tree essential oil to the affected area. For boils, genital herpes, or other external sores, after a bath or shower, apply a single drop of tea tree essential oil directly to the lesion until it disappears.

Blends well with: lavender, lavandin, clary sage, pine, marjoram, rosemary, clove, nutmeg, and other spice oils.

Caution: Tea tree oil can be irritating to sensitive skin.

Thyme *(Thymus vulgaris)*

Thyme essential oil, which is extracted by steam-distillation of the flowering tops of branches, has an intense, herbal aroma. Thyme has been a popular herb since the days of antiquity, a favorite of Egyptians, Greeks, and Romans alike. Thyme essential oil as used in medicinal preparations can be traced to sixteenth-century writings.

Thyme oil is used to treat many emotional and physical ailments, including stress, anxiety, tension, mental fatigue, insomnia, depression, athlete's foot, sinus headaches, colds, asthma, bladder infections, infectious diseases, viruses, lung ailments, rheumatism, inflammation of the skin, and even snakebites (it contains an antivenom agent). Thyme oil is also said to stimulate white blood cell production, accelerate the healing process, and strengthen the immune system. It revives the liver and circulatory system, regulates digestion, and eases indigestion. It is also a disinfectant and insect repellent. This oil is a general stimulant, an antispasmodic, antiseptic, antibiotic, diuretic, and an expectorant. Folklore reveals that thyme brings about courage and confidence.

Recommended use: Blend thyme with frankincense and hyssop for use in a simmer pot or diffuser blend to help refresh a room.

Blends well with: frankincense, hyssop, bergamot, lemon, rosemary, melissa, lavender, lavandin, marjoram, and pine.

Caution: Use in moderation (only a drop or two), as thyme is a very potent essential oil. Overuse is said to stimulate the thyroid gland and the lymphatic system. Never apply thyme oil undiluted directly to the skin. This oil should not be used on children. Avoid during to pregnancy, or if suffering from epilepsy, hyperthyroidism, or high blood pressure.

Tonka Bean *(Dipteryx odorata)*

Tonka bean essential oil is produced through solvent extraction, using benzene or alcohol, from the dried bean. Tonka is a member of the legume family, and most of the beans used for extraction come from South America. Liquids or absolutes are also produced from the solid (concrete). Its aroma is rich, sweet, and somewhat like hay. Tonka bean is known to be uplifting and calming. It is often used in blends for perfumes, but also in massage oils and bath oils. Depending on the other oils you mix with tonka bean, it can create a sensual, euphoric, or relaxing experience. Tonka bean seems to produce an antidepressant effect, especially when mixed with vanilla and geranium oils. It can also be used to combat the symptoms of PMS. Tonka bean can be used as an insecticide, a cardiac tonic, and even a narcotic.

Recommended use: To combat symptoms of PMS, use a few drops of tonka bean in a bath combined with grapefruit, Roman chamomile, and neroli.

Blends well with: clary sage, bergamot, lavender, lavandin, rose, myrtle, vanilla, geranium, jasmine, patchouli, and ylang-ylang.

Caution: Do not take tonka bean internally. Do not use tonka in large doses. It can be a skin irritant.

Tuberose *(Polianthes tuberosa)*

This essential oil, which is extracted with solvents and through enfleurage of the fresh flowers, is one of the most expensive essential oils around; according to some sources, one pound costs about $10,000. In fact, only a little more than thirty pounds of tuberose oil is produced worldwide annually. The oil (actually an absolute) comes from the wild flower from the East Indies, considered one of the sweeter fragrant flowers. It grows from a bulb that is planted in autumn and flowers the following spring. It is said to produce only two full-blown flowers a day, which, if they are to be used to produce essential oil, must be gathered immediately upon opening. Known sometimes as mistress of the night, tuberose has a spicy/flowery aroma and is said to be an aphrodisiac, awakening erotic feelings and attracting romance. Some say that tuberose enhances one's capacity for emotional depth, and it is able to bring peace to the mind and to the heart. Tuberose is considered a tonic for the reproductive system, but it is used mainly for perfume.

Recommended use: The principal use of tuberose is in perfumery, but for a diffuser blend, try mixing 2 drops each of tuberose and ylang-ylang with 5 or 6 drops of sandalwood.

Blends well with: violet, chamomile, lavender, rose, jasmine, myrtle, neroli, patchouli, cumin, and ylang-ylang.

Caution: Do not take internally, as it may be toxic.

Valerian *(Valeriana fauriei)*

The essential oil of valerian is extracted by steam-distillation of the rhizomes. There is also an absolute that is produced by solvent extraction of the rhizomes. The herb is currently cultivated for its oil primarily in Belgium. Its main therapeutic use is to treat disorders of the nervous system, including insomnia, tension, restlessness, migraine headaches, and nervous indigestion. The herb has been used since medieval times (it was called all heal) for its relaxing properties.

Recommended use: Use in a diffuser to combat nervousness or insomnia. You can also add about 5 drops to a warm bath.

Blends well with: lavender, cedarwood, mandarin, pine, patchouli, and rosemary.
   Caution: Valerian can possibly cause skin sensitization and should be used sparingly.

Vanilla *(Vanilla planifolia)*

Vanilla essential oil is extracted with a solvent, usually alcohol, from the pod of a creeper in the orchid family that grows best in Mexico. One of the most popular scents, almost everyone likes vanilla's sweet, mellow aroma. It is considered a relaxing oil, one that cannot only enhance romance, but also can help retain childhood memories (perhaps because it reminds so many of us of home-baked goods). This calming oil is believed to reduce feelings of anger and irritability. Essential oil of vanilla can also act as a stimulant for menstruation.

This soothing, delicious, and familiar scent can overwhelm a blend, so it's good to work with it in small quantities. Vanilla oil is an ingredient used in many types of aromatherapy blends, including body lotions, bath oils, perfumes, scented candles, and diffuser blends.

Recommended use: Diffuse a few drops of vanilla into a room to create a warm, delicious, comforting atmosphere.

Blends well with: most oils, especially vetiver, sandalwood, benzoin, and spice oils. Note, however, that vanilla tends to sink to the bottom of a blend, so you need to shake the mixture well before using.

  Caution: As tempting as it may be, don't use the pure essential oil for baking. Vanilla extract contains the essential oil combined with alcohol.

Verbena or Lemon Verbena *(Lippia citriodora)*

Verbena essential oil is extracted by steam-distillation of the fragrant, lemony leaves of the lemon verbena bush, a garden plant. This oil is cool and refreshing, and it is used as a purifier, a digestive stimulant, and an antispasmodic. It has a mildly sedative effect, so verbena oil can be useful in treating insomnia. The true lemon verbena essential oil is very expensive, but most of what is on the market has been compromised by the addition of lemongrass oil.

Recommended use: For a relaxing, sedative bath, try two drops of verbena oil combined with four drops of lavender. Mix very well. It is recommended to dilute this in another carrier since verbena can be irritating to the skin. Place one or two drops of verbena oil on a cotton ball or tissue and inhale the aroma to relieve nausea and dizziness.

Blends well with: neroli, jasmine, sweet orange, juniper, hyssop, myrtle, tonka bean, and cedarwood.

Caution: Do not use more than two drops of verbena oil in a bath. It is irritating to the skin. Do not use it during pregnancy, except possibly during childbirth to help with contractions.

Note: Much of the lemon verbena being sold today has been adulterated with lemongrass oil, so naturally its effects would be diminished.

Vetiver or Vetivert *(Vetivera zizanioides)*

The essential oil of vetiver is extracted by steam-distillation from the roots of vetiver, a wild grass that grows in Indonesia and the Philippines, as well as India, Ceylon, Japan, and other places around the world such as South America and the Caribbean. This essence has an earthy-woody, smoky aroma and a sweet undertone. Vetiver has a long history of being used in perfumes. The aroma, some say, is more pleasant when diluted. Vetiver is a polarizing oil; you either love it or hate it.

This essential oil is considered soothing and deeply relaxing for the mind and body. It helps to reduce high blood pressure and can be used to treat nervous tension and stress, exhaustion, and even anorexia. Known as a grounding oil, its aroma can be helpful when we find ourselves under stress and our emotions run wild. Believed to be a centering and nurturing oil, vetiver is recommended for times when feelings of insecurity surface.

It reportedly stimulates circulation and helps relieve arthritis and joint pain. It also has sensual properties (if you're among those who like the scent), considered to be an oil that awakens sexuality and repels negativity. Men find it particularly appealing. It has a regenerative effect on skin, especially for acne, cuts and wounds, and for oily skin. In the East, the essence is known as the oil of tranquillity, and is often used in meditation. According to legend, vetiver is supposed to bring protection and attract prosperity and love.

Recommended use: Combine two or three drops of vetiver in 3½ ounces of massage oil for dealing with exhaustion. Vetiver can also be used in an aroma lamp or diffuser.

Blends well with: lavender, clary sage, ylang-ylang, orange, lemon verbena, mimosa, geranium, rose, neroli, tuberose, tonka bean, sandalwood, and jasmine.

Violet *(Viola odorata)*

The essential oil (actually an absolute) comes from the leaf and the flowers via solvent extraction. It is grown mainly in Grasse in southern France. The violet leaf absolute is more common, but it is still relatively rare in use for aromatherapy. It is more often an ingredient in perfumery, and it is very expensive. The leaf absolute has a dry, haylike aroma with a floral undertone. The flower absolute has a sweeter floral aroma. The flowers are used to make a syrup of violet, which is still used for its laxative qualities and as a coloring agent. Violet is an antiseptic and is beneficial in the treatment of skin conditions, including acne, eczema, and in healing wounds. Violet has painkilling properties. It is also considered useful in treating conditions of the nervous system, including dizziness, nervous exhaustion, and insomnia. Napoleon reportedly wrote notes to Josephine on violet-scented paper. This was a very popular scent in Victorian times.

Recommended use: Add a few drops of violet leaf oil to a facial oil or a facial steam bath to help combat wrinkles.

Blends well with: tuberose, clary sage, tarragon, cumin, basil, and other floral oils.

Caution: May cause sensitization in some people.

Yarrow *(Achillea millefolium)*

This warm, aromatic, camphorlike essential oil is steam-distilled from the dried herb or flowering plant, which can be found in Europe and Asia. It has sedative properties, which make it useful for treating nervous exhaustion, insomnia, and other stress-related conditions. Considered good for bringing about a quick recovery from the flu and for healing all mucous membranes, yarrow is also used for a wide variety of ailments, including toothaches, chest infections, colds, fever, and digestive problems.

The Chinese use it for menstrual problems and hemorrhoids, and in Scandinavia it is used for rheumatism. It is also used for skin problems, including acne, eczema, rashes, varicose veins, and for minimizing scarring from burns or cuts. Its usefulness in caring for injuries, in fact, reportedly dates back to Achilles, who was said to have used yarrow to treat the wounds inflicted by the iron weapons of the time. Yarrow is also known to be anti-inflammatory, antiseptic, antispasmodic, astringent, expectorant, carminative, and tonic.

It is good when used in a shampoo to stimulate hair growth and alleviate dandruff. Yarrow can reportedly be used to help stop internal and external bleeding, since it helps blood to thicken. Legend has it that yarrow attracts love and serenity, as well as self-confidence and courage.

Recommended use: Add equal parts of yarrow and lavender oils (about five drops each) to a spray bottle filled with water (approximately four ounces). Spray on sunburned skin for relief.

Blends well with: balm, cedarwood, chamomile, lavender, clary sage, hyssop, pine, and myrtle.

Caution: Those with skin sensitivities should use yarrow essential oil with caution, as it can cause irritation when exposed to sunlight.

*Ylang-ylang *(Cananga odorata)*

Ylang-ylang, known as the flower of flowers, produces a sweet, exotic floral oil that is extracted by the steam-distillation of fresh flowers. Cultivated today in Madagascar and Haiti, among other places, the ylang-ylang tree originated in the Philippines. Just like rose and jasmine blossoms, ylang-ylang blossoms must be harvested and prepared in the early-morning hours in order to capture the highest-quality essence.

Ylang-ylang has many healing properties, including anti-depressant, aphrodisiac, sedative, anti-infectious, and anti-septic. Many claim it induces a sense of euphoria. It is useful in treating acne, irritated, dry, or oily skin, and for general care for all skin types. It also is good for helping hair growth, as well as a hair rinse (try two drops in a rinse water). It is also useful for treating insect bites and high blood pressure. It balances hormones and is a sedative for rapid breathing, rapid heartbeat, or palpitations.* This soothing and relaxing oil helps fight depression, frigidity, impotence, insomnia, nervous tension, and other stress-related disorders, including anger and anxiety. An evening bath ex-

*If you are experiencing heart irregularities, you should immediately seek medical attention.

perience with ylang-ylang is very useful for easing the pressures of the day. It is great for PMS, especially in combination with clary sage and neroli oils in a diffuser or in a bath or body oil.

Ylang-ylang has long been used for its sensual properties. It is great in massage oils and in perfumes. You either love ylang-ylang right away, or it literally gives you a headache. Often called "the poor person's jasmine," ylang-ylang has a lingering effect that even allows other oils that it is mixed with to maintain their fragrance longer. Ylang-ylang is, in fact, frequently used in fragrances.

Recommended use: Use two drops of ylang-ylang oil in a diffuser to calm nerves and create a romantic atmosphere. For a relaxing bath, try two drops of ylang-ylang, two drops of rose, and three or four drops of lavender. A couple of drops of patchouli could also be added.

Blends well with: rosewood, lavender, sandalwood, lemon, orange, bergamot, mimosa, jasmine, neroli, tonka bean, patchouli, vetiver, rose, and tuberose, among others.

Caution: Ylang-ylang may cause skin sensitization in some people.

CHAPTER 4

Choosing an Essential Oil

Choosing an essential oil is really based on individual choice. It's part intuition, part preference, and part therapy. There are many different reasons for choosing an essential oil. Perhaps you are attracted to a particular aroma, or maybe you need to balance your mood or emotional state. Sometimes you are in need of something with specific healing abilities.

While this and other books on the subject of aromatherapy and essential oils go into great detail about which oil to use for what situation, it's really up to you and your aromatherapy practitioner to determine what works best for you and under what conditions.

Often your body will tell you what essence is right for you. Through sensory testing, you can sometimes just know what will work. You will naturally be attracted or repelled by certain oils based on your memories, your mood, and your own body chemistry. Just as two people may not interpret a film the same way, essential oils, while possessing certain properties, won't affect everyone the same way. The same person may even have different reactions to the same oil at different times. You might always love the smell of geranium, for example, but there might be times when even a favorite scent will be a turn-off. Listen to your body. It usually knows best.

Despite the fickle nature of the human body, however, there are some general beliefs about how most people will *usually* respond to various oils. A lot of this is based on anecdotal information and some scientific evidence, widely acknowledged by aromatherapy experts. Essential oils can be used as singular notes or in blends with other essential oils and/or carriers. What follows is a compilation of this information.

Experimentation with care is my best recommendation.

These recommendations use the common names of the essential oils. In most cases, however, there are many varieties of each botanical species. The oils derived from the different varieties will often have different properties and therefore somewhat different therapeutic uses.

The suggestions here can be used as a general guide but are by no means exhaustive. For other recommendations, consult a qualified aromatherapy practitioner or refer to the many fine books available on the subject of aromatherapy.

What follows is intended as a basic summary of available options. Many symptoms are indicative of more serious illness, so it is always advisable to seek professional medical advice when you are ill. Often, to properly treat an ailment, you will need to identify the cause. Aromatherapy is a complement to other medical treatment, not a substitute.

THERAPEUTIC USES FOR ESSENTIAL OILS

Abdominal Cramps

Most useful: basil, melissa

Also try: aniseed, bergamot, caraway, clove, fennel, marjoram, neroli, nutmeg

Recommended application: massage, compress, bath

Abrasions

Most useful: lavender

Also try: tea tree, neroli, frankincense, myrrh

Recommended application: soak, neat application (lavender, possibly tea tree)

Add five drops of lavender to a bowl of warm water. With sterile cotton or gauze, use this water mixture to clean the affected area. Then apply one drop of lavender onto the abrasion.

Abscesses

See also **boils.**

Most useful: bergamot, chamomile, immortelle, lavender, tea tree

Also try: eucalyptus, clove, lavandin, lemon, niaouli, clary sage, thyme

Recommended application: oil/lotion, compress, bath

Acne

Most useful: bergamot, chamomile, geranium, juniper, lavender, lemon, palmarosa, rosemary, tea tree

Also try: camphor, cedarwood, clary sage, clove bud, cypress, eucalyptus, grapefruit, lavandin, lemongrass, lime, mandarin, peppermint, myrrh, myrtle, niaouli, patchouli, petitgrain, rosewood, sage, sandalwood, thyme, vetiver, violet, yarrow, ylang-ylang

Recommended application: massage, lotion/oil, flower water, bath, inhalation/steam, neat application (lavender, possibly tea tree or eucalyptus)

Using a cotton swab, apply a lavender, tea tree, or eucalyptus on a pimple overnight.

Air Disinfectant

Most useful: pine, eucalyptus

Also try: grapefruit, lemon, sage

Recommended application: diffusion, room spray

Allergies and Hay Fever

Most useful: lavender

Also try: hyssop, chamomile, eucalyptus

Recommended application: oil/lotion, inhalation, vaporization

Blend one drop of lavender essential oil into one teaspoon

of carrier oil/lotion. Once a day, massage the blend into the skin over the sinuses around the nose.

Put two drops of hyssop on a tissue or handkerchief and inhale. Also use hyssop in a vaporizer or blend with a carrier lotion and use for a facial massage.

Allergies, Skin

Most useful: chamomile, lavender

Also try: melissa

Recommended application: massage, oil/lotion, flower water, bath, inhalation/steam

Alopecia

Most useful: lavender, rosemary, thyme

Also try: carrot, sage

Recommended application: hair rinse, massage

Anger

Most useful: rose

Also try: benzoin, chamomile, cedarwood, clary sage

Recommended application: inhalation, bath, oil/lotion, diffuser

Anxiety and Tension

Most useful: lavender, clary, geranium, ylang-ylang, bergamot, melissa

Also try: basil, cedarwood, chamomile (Roman), lemon, marjoram, myrrh, neroli, patchouli, petitgrain, rose, sweet thyme, vetiver

Recommended application: diffuser, bath, massage oil, vaporization, steam inhalation

Use a few drops of lavender essential oil in a bath or add lavender oil to a basin of steaming (not boiling) water; cover your head and the basin with a towel and breathe in slowly and deeply.

Caution: Asthma sufferers should not use steam inhalation. Instead, put two or three drops of the essential oil on a tissue or handkerchief and inhale the aroma as necessary.

Appendicitis

Most useful: lavender

Recommended application: compress

Note: This is a first aid remedy only. Serious conditions should be treated by a medical professional.

Appetite, Loss of

Most useful: bergamot, coriander

Also try: chamomile (Roman), cardamom, fennel, ginger, mandarin, myrrh, black pepper

Recommended application: massage

Arthritis

Most useful: benzoin, rosemary, chamomile, black pepper, cajeput, eucalyptus, ginger, juniper, lemon, sage, (sweet) thyme

Also try: clove, coriander, cypress, frankincense, lavender, marjoram, yarrow, myrrh

Recommended application: massage, bath, oil/lotion, compress

Asthma

Most useful: Aniseed, clary sage, frankincense, melissa, peppermint, sage

Also try: benzoin, cajeput, chamomile (Roman), clove bud, cypress, eucalyptus, hyssop, immortelle, lavandin, lemon, lime, sweet marjoram, myrrh, myrtle, niaouli, rosemary, tea tree, thyme

Recommended application: massage, vaporization, inhalation (dry—do not use steam if you are suffering from asthma)

Athlete's Foot

Most useful: lavender, myrrh, tea tree, pine

Also try: clove bud, eucalyptus, lemon, lemongrass, patchouli, peppermint

Recommended application: oil/lotion, footbath, neat application (lavender, possibly tea tree)

Backache

Most useful: chamomile, white birch, rosemary, coriander, eucalyptus, ginger, black pepper, lavender

Also try: thyme, peppermint, rosemary, juniper

Recommended application: massage, compress

Bad Breath

See **Halitosis.**

Baldness/Hair Care

Most useful: bay, chamomile, rosemary, yarrow

Also try: white birch, cedarwood, clary sage, grapefruit, juniper, patchouli, sage, ylang-ylang

Recommended application: lotion, hair rinse, shampoo, massage

Bee Stings

Most useful: chamomile

Recommended application: compress

Apply a few drops of chamomile oil to a clean, damp cloth or cotton pad. Use on the affected area three times daily for a two-day period.

Blisters

Most useful: bergamot, chamomile, geranium, lavender, tea tree

Also try: eucalyptus, immortelle, lavandin, lemon, niaouli, clary sage, thyme

Recommended application: lotion, compress, bath

Boils

Most useful: bergamot, chamomile, lavender, tea tree

Also try: eucalyptus, immortelle, lavandin, lemon, niaouli, clary sage, thyme

Recommended application: lotion, compress, bath, neat application (lavender, possibly tea tree)
   Soak a cotton compress in hot water and a few drops of chamomile oil. Apply to the boil and leave on until the compress cools.

Breast-Feeding Problems

Most useful: fennel

Recommended application: massage oil

Brittle Nails

Most useful: bay, lavender, myrrh, sandalwood

Also try: cypress

Recommended application: massage oil, soak

Bronchitis

Most useful: aniseed, basil, benzoin, bergamot, eucalyptus, frankincense, sweet marjoram, myrrh, myrtle, niaouli, sandalwood

Also try: angelica, cajeput, camphor (white), cardamom, cedarwood, clove bud, cypress, hyssop, immortelle, lavandin, lavender, lemon, melissa, peppermint, orange (bitter and sweet), pine, rosemary, sage, sandalwood, tea tree, thyme, violet

Recommended application: massage, vaporization, inhalation/steam

Bruises

Most useful: camphor, chamomile (German), fennel, geranium, hyssop, lavender

Also try: clove bud, rosemary, sweet marjoram, thyme

Recommended application: oil/lotion, compress, neat application (lavender)

Burns

Most useful: lavender (spike and true)

Also try: benzoin, chamomile, clove bud, eucalyptus, geranium, immortelle, lavandin, marigold, niaouli, tea tree, yarrow

Recommended application: compress, neat application (lavender)

Apply a drop or two of lavender directly to the wound after it is cleaned thoroughly.

Cool the burn in cold water for at least ten minutes. Soak a sterile gauze in ice water. Add any of the recommended essential oils listed on the previous page (approximately one drop per square inch of affected skin area) and apply to the burn. (Note: Lavender oil, an antibiotic, is especially helpful in reducing the risk of infection related to a burn.)

Candida (Thrush)

Most useful: tea tree, thyme

Also try: bergamot, cinnamon, eucalyptus, rosemary, rose (otto), rosewood

Recommended application: sitz bath

For a sitz bath, add three or four drops of tea tree to a bowl or shallow tub of warm water. Sit in it for ten minutes.

Catarrh (Inflammation of Mucous Membranes)

Most useful: eucalyptus, lavender, marjoram, peppermint, pine, tea tree, thyme

Also try: benzoin, black pepper, cajeput, cedarwood, frankincense, ginger, hyssop, jasmine, lavandin, lemon, lime, myrrh, myrtle, niaouli, rosemary, sandalwood, violet

Recommended application: massage, vaporization, inhalation/steam

Cellulitis

Most useful: white birch, sweet fennel, geranium, grape-fruit, juniper

Also try: cypress, lemon, parsley, rosemary, thyme

Recommended application: massage, lotion, bath

Chapped Lips

Most useful: chamomile, geranium

Recommended application: oil/lotion, gel
    Mix two drops of chamomile, two drops of geranium, and two teaspoons of aloe vera gel. Apply to chapped lips.

Chapped Skin

Most useful: benzoin, lavender, myrrh, patchouli, rose

Also try: sandalwood, neroli

Recommended application: lotion/oil, flower water, bath
    For very chapped skin, try six drops of lavender, six drops of sandalwood, and six drops of rose in four ounces of carrier oil made of two ounces of soy oil, one ounce of almond oil, one ounce of avocado oil, and one tablespoon of wheat germ oil.*

Chicken Pox

Most useful: true lavender, tea tree

*Adapted from Judith Jackson, p. 196.

Also try: bergamot, chamomile, eucalyptus, lemon

Recommended application: compress, lotion/oil, bath

To lessen the possibility of scarring, use ten drops of tea tree, ten drops of lavender, and five drops of lemon blended with two tablespoons of carrier oil. Apply to the rash several times a day. Don't keep this blend for more than five days, as it will spoil.

Chills

Most useful: black pepper, cinnamon leaf, geranium, ginger

Also try: benzoin, camphor (white), grapefruit, orange (bitter and sweet)

Recommended application: massage, bath

Chronic Coughs

See also Coughs.

Most useful: frankincense, hyssop, myrtle

Also try: lemon balm, benzoin, cypress, immortelle, jasmine, myrrh, peppermint, sandalwood

Recommended application: massage, vaporization, inhalation/steam

Cold Sores (Fever Blisters)

Most useful: bergamot, eucalyptus, geranium, melissa, rose, tea tree

Also try: lemon, lavender, myrrh

Recommended application: oil/lotion, neat application (lavender, which is soothing; possibly tea tree)

Apply a single drop of tea tree oil twice a day, once in the morning and again at bedtime. (Note: Some aromatherapists say that you can use geranium or eucalyptus every hour.)

Blend together a small amount of tea tree, bergamot, lavender, and geranium into a ⅟₁₆-ounce amber bottle. Apply a drop of the blend directly to the cold sore.

Colds

See **Common Cold.**

Colic

Most useful: chamomile, lavender, sweet marjoram, peppermint

Also try: aniseed, black pepper, cardamom, carrot seed, clary sage, clove bud, coriander, cumin, dill, sweet fennel, ginger, hyssop, immortelle, lavandin, orange blossom, parsley, rosemary

Recommended application: massage

Common Cold

Most useful: eucalyptus, ginger, thyme, lemon, rosemary, tea tree

Also try: lavender, clove, peppermint

Recommended application: bath, steam inhalation, diffusion, massage

Using steam inhalation, use one drop each of thyme, tea

tree, lavender, and clove (or use one drop each of tea tree and lemon). Add to a basin of steaming (not boiling) water, cover your head and the basin with a towel, and breathe in slowly and deeply.

To relieve chest congestion, use steam inhalation as above, with one or two drops of eucalyptus or peppermint.

Caution: Asthma sufferers should not use steam inhalation. Instead, put two or three drops of the essential oil on a tissue or handkerchief and inhale the aroma as necessary.

Congestion

See also **Common Cold.**

Most useful: eucalyptus, pine, myrtle, niaouli, lemon

Also try: peppermint, frankincense

Recommended application: vaporization, inhalation/steam

Mix two drops of eucalyptus, one drop of peppermint, and one drop of frankincense in a steam inhalation.

Caution: Asthma sufferers should not use steam inhalation. Instead, put two or three drops of the essential oil on a tissue or handkerchief and inhale the aroma as necessary.

Conjunctivitis

Most useful: chamomile

Recommended application: compress

Although some aromatherapy sources say you can use chamomile essential oil in a compress on the eyes, many others agree that any contact of essential oils with the eyes is a bad idea. A recommended alternative is to use strong chamomile tea. Make the tea as directed and let it cool so that it's lukewarm. Use the tea as an eyewash or on a compress. If you make the tea from tea bags, you can even place the cooled tea bags over the eyes as a compress. It feels great, and it really works. You can use this treatment for other types of eye inflammation, such as allergic reactions, in combination with a treatment of plain hot compresses (for three to four minutes) followed by a cold compress for about twenty to thirty seconds. Do this several times a day.

Constipation

Most useful: black pepper, peppermint, rosemary, thyme

Also try: basil, chamomile (Roman), cinnamon leaf, coriander, sweet fennel, ginger, lavage, sweet marjoram, nutmeg, orange (bitter and sweet), palmarosa, pine, tarragon, yarrow

Recommended application: bath, massage

Coughs

See also **Chronic Coughs.**

Most useful: benzoin, cedarwood, clary sage, eucalyptus, hyssop, sweet marjoram, pine, sage, and thyme

Also try: angelica, aniseed, black pepper, cajeput, camphor (white), caraway, ginger, myrrh, niaouli, rose, rosemary, rockrose, tea tree

Recommended application: massage, vaporization, inhalation/ steam

Remember Vicks VapoRub? This product is basically a decongestant made from eucalyptus. To make your own version, combine three drops of eucalyptus oil, two drops of thyme oil, and two teaspoons of carrier oil. Massage this into the chest and neck regions.

Cramp

Most useful: basil, chamomile, sweet marjoram, rosemary

Also try: ginger, geranium, cajeput, cypress, lavender, valerian

Recommended application: compress, massage

Cuts/Sores

See also **Wounds.**

Most useful: chamomile, geranium, lavender, marigold, rosemary, tea tree, yarrow

Also try: benzoin, bergamot, clove bud, eucalyptus, hyssop, immortelle, lavandin, lemon, lime, myrrh, niaouli, orange (bitter), pine, sage, thyme, vetiver

Recommended application: oil/lotion, compress

Cystitis

Most useful: bergamot, chamomile, juniper, lavender, sandalwood

Also try: basil (sweet), cajeput, cedarwood, clove, coriander, eucalyptus, frankincense, hyssop, jasmine, peppermint, niaouli, thyme, tea tree

Recommended application: bath

Add five or six drops of bergamot to a warm bath and soak for ten to fifteen minutes.

Dandruff

Most useful: bay, lavender, rosemary

Also try: cedarwood, clary sage, cypress, eucalyptus, lemon, patchouli, peppermint, sage, tea tree

Recommended application: shampoo, rinse, hair oil

Depression

Most useful: basil, bergamot, chamomile, camphor, clary, geranium, hyssop, jasmine, lavender, melissa, neroli, patchouli, petitgrain, pine, rose, sandalwood, thyme, ylang-ylang

Also try: cinnamon bark, cypress, frankincense, juniper, marjoram (sweet), niaouli, rosemary, rosewood, vetiver

Recommended application: inhalation, bath, massage

Try a massage or bath using a combination of either basil and neroli or marjoram and ylang-ylang. For massage, use six drops of each oil blended with four ounces of carrier oil. For a warm bath, use twenty drops of each. Soak in the tub for ten minutes.

As with all essential oil treatments, the results will be individual, based on a person's likes and dislikes. When choosing an oil as an antidepressant, make sure it's one that gives you pleasure.

Dermatitis

Most useful: bergamot, chamomile, lavender, melissa, neroli

Also try: benzoin, white birch, carrot seed, cedarwood, clary sage, geranium, hyssop, immortelle, juniper, palmarosa, patchouli, peppermint, rose otto, sage, thyme

Recommended application: oil/lotion, compress, flower water, bath

Add 5 drops of chamomile (Roman) to a warm bath. Soak for approximately ten minutes before bedtime.

Diarrhea

Most useful: ginger, lavender, chamomile, peppermint

Also try: benzoin, black pepper, cypress, eucalyptus, fennel, neroli

Recommended application: massage

Drowsiness

Most useful: rosemary, basil

Also try: eucalyptus, geranium, peppermint

Recommended application: diffusion, inhalation

Dry, Sensitive Skin

Most useful: chamomile, jasmine, geranium, lavender, rose, sandalwood, ylang-ylang

Also try: cedarwood, frankincense, lavandin, neroli, rosewood, violet

Recommended application: massage, oil/lotion, flower water, bath

Dry, Itchy Eyes

Most useful: tea tree

Recommended application: humidifier

Dull Skin

Most useful: angelica, geranium, grapefruit, lavender, rosemary

Also try: white birch, sweet fennel, lavandin, lemon, lime, mandarin, peppermint, myrtle, niaouli, orange (bitter and sweet), palmarosa, rose, rosewood, ylang-ylang

Recommended application: massage, oil/lotion, flower water, bath, inhalation/steam

Earache

Most useful: chamomile, lavender

Also try: basil, cajeput, rosemary

Recommended application: compress

Eczema

Most useful: bergamot, chamomile, immortelle, lavender, patchouli, rose

Also try: white birch, carrot seed, cedarwood, geranium, hyssop, juniper, lavandin, marigold, melissa, myrrh, rosemary, sage, thyme, violet, yarrow

Recommended application: massage, lotion, flower water, bath

Emphysema

Most useful: eucalyptus

Recommended application: inhalation, vaporization

Fatigue

Most useful: rosemary, geranium, basil

Also try: orange (sweet), mandarin, peppermint, juniper, lavender

Recommended application: bath, inhalation, diffusion

Put a drop each of rosemary and basil on a tissue or handkerchief and inhale the aroma to combat feelings of fatigue. Also substitute geranium for the rosemary.

For a bath, use ten drops of juniper and ten drops of lavender in a tub of warm water. Soak for ten minutes. Also try a bath with ten drops of rosemary and ten drops of geranium. These combinations are also great in a footbath. Use two quarts of warm water and ten drops each of the two essential oils.

In a room diffuser, use four drops of rosemary and two drops of sweet orange or mandarin. This blend will keep you awake but calm, so it's better than a cup of coffee.

Fever

Most useful: eucalyptus, peppermint, rosemary, tea tree, yarrow

Also try: basil, bergamot, camphor (white), ginger, immortelle, juniper, lemon, lemongrass, lime, myrtle, niaouli, rosewood, sage, thyme

Recommended application: compress, bath
   Add ten drops of eucalyptus and ten drops of lavender to one quart of cool water. After mixing well, place a small compress into the water. Alternate the compress between the forehead and the chest, making sure to soak the compress in the water mixture as needed. Repeat several times. A soothing compress can also be made by using twenty drops of peppermint oil.

Flatulence/Indigestion

Most useful: aniseed, bergamot, black pepper, camphor, caraway, cardamom, chamomile, clary sage, coriander, sweet fennel, hyssop, juniper, lavender, sweet marjoram, peppermint, myrrh, orange (bitter and sweet), rosemary

Also try: angelica, basil, black pepper, carrot seed, cinnamon leaf, clary sage, clove bud, coriander, cumin, eucalyptus, ginger, hyssop, lavandin, lemongrass, melissa, myrrh, nutmeg, orange blossom, parsley, thyme, yarrow

Recommended application: massage

Foot Odor

Most useful: cypress, lemon

Recommended application: footbath

Frigidity

Most useful: orange blossom, patchouli, rose, ylang-ylang

Also try: cinnamon (leaf), jasmine, nutmeg, black pepper, rosewood, clary sage, sandalwood

Recommended application: massage, oil/lotion, bath, vaporization

Gastroenteritis

Most useful: cajeput, chamomile, juniper, niaouli, peppermint

Also try: bergamot, caraway, clove, coriander, cypress, fennel, lavandin, lemongrass, mandarin, sweet marjoram, nutmeg, patchouli, sage, tea tree

Recommended application: massage, oil/lotion

Gingivitis

Most useful: tea tree

Recommended application: dental hygiene
   Add a drop of tea tree essential oil to your toothbrush (on top of toothpaste) and brush as usual.

Gout

Most useful: juniper, rosemary

Also try: basil, chamomile, fennel, lemon, pine

Recommended application: massage, oil/lotion, footbath

Make a massage oil of five drops of juniper essential oil and one ounce of olive oil. Use several times daily.

Use ten drops of juniper and ten drops of rosemary in two quarts of cool water for a footbath.

Greasy/Oily Skin or Scalp

Most useful: bergamot, cypress, geranium, lavender, sandalwood, tea tree

Also try: cajeput, camphor (white), carrot seed, fennel, jasmine, juniper, lemon, lemongrass, mandarin, marigold, myrtle, niaouli, palmarosa, patchouli, petitgrain, rosemary, rosewood, clary sage, thyme, vetivert, ylang-ylang

Recommended application: oil/lotion, hair rinse, shampoo

Grief (Sorrow)

Most useful: marjoram, rose otto

Also try: bergamot, benzoin, chamomile, clary sage, eucalyptus, frankincense, juniper, lavender, mandarin, melissa, niaouli, orange (bitter), petitgrain, rosewood, thyme, ylang-ylang

Recommended application: inhalation

Put one to two drops of marjoram on a tissue. Inhale as needed.

Halitosis (Bad Breath)

Most useful: cardamom, sweet fennel, grapefruit, peppermint, myrrh

Also try: bergamot, lavandin, lavender

Recommended application: oil/lotion, neat application
Try a drop of pure peppermint essential oil on the tongue.

Headache

See also **Migraine.**

Most useful: chamomile, lavender, peppermint

Also try: citronella, clary sage, eucalyptus, grapefruit, lavandin, lemongrass, sweet marjoram, rose, rosemary, rosewood, sage, thyme, violet

Recommended application: massage, oil/lotion, compress, inhalation, vaporization, neat application (lavender)
Add a drop of peppermint essential oil to unscented lotion. Apply under the nose and behind the ear. Also, try inhaling it directly from the bottle.

Place one to two drops of lavender oil on your fingertips. Massage, using a circular motion, across the temples, the sides of your eyes, behind the ears, and across the back of your neck.

Caution: Be sure your fingers do not get too close to your eyes.

Try twenty drops of lavender or peppermint (or other oil mentioned above) in a bowl filled with one quart of hot (not boiling) water. Place a towel over your head and inhale the steam. Avoid steam inhalation if your suffer from asthma.

For any type of headache, try: *Compress:* two drops of peppermint oil on a compress for your forehead. *Bath:* five drops of peppermint oil in a bath.

For neck tension or eyestrain headache, try: *Compress:*

two drops of lavender oil on a compress for your forehead. *Bath:* three drops of lavender oil in a bath.

For gastric or nervous-tension headache, try: *Compress:* two drops of chamomile oil on a compress for your forehead. *Bath:* five drops of chamomile oil in a bath.

Headache bath hint: Before getting into your bath, massage a couple of drops of lavender oil into the back of your neck. While you're soaking in your hot bath, place an ice compress on your forehead or wrap a towel filled with ice around your head.

Heartburn

Most useful: black pepper

Also try: cardamom

Recommended application: massage

Heat Exhaustion

Most useful: lavender, eucalyptus

Recommended application: neat application, compress

Hemorrhoids

Most useful: chamomile, clary, cypress, juniper, lavender, myrrh, neroli, niaouli, peppermint, yarrow

Also try: coriander, geranium, lavender, myrtle, parsley, sandalwood, tea tree

Recommended application: lotion, compress, bath/sitz bath
    For a sitz bath, add two drops of cypress and one drop of

peppermint to a bowl or shallow bath of warm water. Sit for ten minutes. Cypress and chamomile make another good combination. Then combine two drops of lavender and one drop of geranium. Blend with one ounce of carrier oil. Apply to affected area after the sitz bath and after every bowel movement.

Hiccups

Most useful: fennel, mandarin

Also try: chamomile, lemon

Recommended application: steam inhalation or inhale neat from the bottle

High Blood Pressure/Hypertension

Most useful: garlic, true lavender, sweet marjoram, yarrow, ylang-ylang

Also try: clary sage, lemon, melissa

Recommended application: massage, bath, vaporization

Hysteria

Most useful: basil, chamomile, clary sage, hyssop, lavender, lemongrass, marjoram, melissa, neroli

Also try: camphor, peppermint, rosemary

Recommended application: inhalation

Impotence

Most useful: ginger, patchouli, sandalwood, clary sage, ylang-ylang

Also try: aniseed, black pepper, cinnamon (bark), peppermint, pine (said to stimulate sperm production), rose otto, thyme (sweet)

Recommended application: massage oil, diffusion, inhalation

Make a massage oil with six drops of patchouli and six drops of sandalwood blended into four ounces of carrier oil.

Also try clary sage and ylang-ylang blended and burned as a room fragrance.

Indigestion

Most useful: aniseed, black pepper, peppermint, chamomile, ginger, lavender, marjoram, melissa

Also try: coriander, fennel, basil, rosemary, dill, orange (sweet), lemongrass

Recommended application: bath, massage, compress

Infections

Most useful: lavender, chamomile, eucalyptus, tea tree

Also try: thyme

Recommended application: compress

Infertility (Female)

Most useful: rose

Also try: chamomile (Roman), clary sage, coriander, cypress, fennel, geranium, nutmeg, thyme

Recommended application: bath, massage

Combine three or four drops of rose oil in ½ ounce of lotion or base oil (jojoba oil will stabilize a base oil if you want to mix up a quantity of the blend). Rub this on your abdomen each day. Many practitioners suggest combining this treatment with meditation and visualization (such as getting pregnant easily, having an easy pregnancy and an easy delivery).

Put three or four drops of rose oil in a warm bath.

Infertility (Male)

Most useful: cedarwood, clary sage, cumin, thyme, vetiver

Also try: angelica, basil

Recommended application: bath, massage

Inflammation

Most useful: chamomile, clary sage, rose

Also try: frankincense, geranium, lavender, myrrh, peppermint (only up to 1 percent), sandalwood

Recommended application: compress, lotion

Influenza

Most useful: eucalyptus, lavender, peppermint, rosemary, tea tree

Also try: black pepper, cypress, hyssop

Recommended application: bath, diffusion

Insect Bites

Most useful: chamomile, immortelle, lavender, melissa, thyme, tea tree

Also try: basil, bergamot, cajeput, cinnamon leaf, eucalyptus, lavandin, lemon, marigold, marjoram, melissa, niaouli, ylang-ylang

Recommended application: oil/lotion, neat application (lavender only)

Mix three drops of lavender and three drops of thyme with two tablespoons of carrier oil. Apply to the affected area.

Also apply lavender neat to the affected area.

Insect Repellent

Most useful: cedarwood, citronella, lavender, lemon, lemongrass, thyme, peppermint

Also try: basil, bergamot, camphor (white), clove, cypress, eucalyptus, geranium, melissa, patchouli, rosemary

Recommended application: oil/lotion, vaporization, room spray

Mix ten drops of lemon and ten drops clove, and blend into four ounces of carrier oil. Apply to bite-prone areas.

Burn one or a combination of these oils in areas that tend to attract insects: lemon and clove, geranium and eucalyptus, or peppermint on its own.

Insomnia

Most useful: lavender, marjoram, ylang-ylang

Also try: chamomile (Roman), melissa, clary sage, lemon, patchouli, neroli, sandalwood, cypress, geranium, valerian

Recommended application: bath, inhalation, diffusion

Add to seven to ten drops of one of the above-mentioned essential oils to a warm bath before bed. Soak for ten minutes.

Apply four drops of lavender, chamomile, or marjoram essential oil to your pillow just before you go to sleep, or put a few drops in a vaporizer. You'll be out in no time.

Make a massage oil formula using ten to twelve drops of any of the above oils in four ounces of carrier oil.

Jet Lag

Most useful: lavender, eucalyptus, peppermint, geranium

Also try: lemongrass, grapefruit, rosemary

Recommended application: compress, bath, inhalation

Put two drops of lavender on a cool, wet washcloth. Wipe your forehead and temples during your flight. Once at your destination, take a bath with ten to fifteen drops of geranium. If you need an extra boost to fight off drowsiness, use rosemary in a diffuser or inhale a couple of drops that have been added to a tissue or handkerchief.

Labor Pains (Childbirth)

Most useful: clary sage, jasmine, lavender, nutmeg, rose

Also try: cinnamon (leaf)

Recommended application: massage, compress, bath, inhalation

Laryngitis/Hoarse Voice

Most useful: benzoin, chamomile, lavender, lemon, peppermint, sandalwood, thyme

Also try: black pepper, cajeput, clary sage, cypress, lemon, eucalyptus, frankincense, geranium, jasmine, lavandin, myrrh, sage

Recommended application: inhalation/steam, gargle
   Combine three drops of lavender, two drops of chamomile, and one drop of thyme. Use this for steam inhalations.
   Gargle with one drop of sandalwood and one drop of lavender in ½ glass of warm water. Add two drops of lemon or peppermint to the gargle if you are fighting an infection.

Leg Cramps

Most useful: lavender

Also try: chamomile, tarragon

Recommended application: massage

Massage four or five drops of lavender, tarragon, or chamomile essential oil directly into the affected area. Dilute these in a carrier oil if you have sensitive skin.

Measles

Most useful: eucalyptus, tea tree

Also try: bergamot, lavender

Recommended application: oil/lotion, bath, inhalation/steam, vaporization

Menopause Problems

Most useful: clary sage, rose, geranium

Also try: chamomile, sage, cypress, fennel, jasmine, lavender

Recommended application: massage, bath, inhalation

Put a drop or two of clary sage essential oil on a tissue or handkerchief. Carry it with you so you can have instant relief from hot flashes wherever you go.

Add twenty drops of cypress or of cypress and lavender to a warm bath. Soak for ten minutes.

Menstrual Cramps

Most useful: chamomile, lavender, sweet marjoram

Also try: cypress, jasmine, lavandin, juniper, rose, rosemary, sage, yarrow

Recommended application: massage, compress, bath

Combine six drops of chamomile and marjoram with four ounces of carrier oil. Massage this into your lower abdomen and lower back.

Mental Fatigue (Weak Memory)

Most useful: rosemary

Also try: petitgrain

Recommended application: inhalation, diffusion

Mental Fatigue (Poor Concentration)

Most useful: basil, cardamom, bergamot, cedarwood, grapefruit, lemon, peppermint, rosemary

Also try: cajeput, clove bud, coriander, cypress, eucalyptus, juniper, melissa, neroli, niaouli, petitgrain, rosewood, sandalwood, thyme

Recommended application: inhalation, diffusion

Migraine

See also **Headache.**

Most useful: lavender, rosemary

Also try: angelica, aniseed, basil, chamomile, citronella, clary sage, coriander, eucalyptus, sweet marjoram, melissa, peppermint, valerian, yarrow

Recommended application: massage, bath, compress, inhalation, diffusion, neat application (lavender only)

Blend ten drops of rosemary and ten drops of chamomile into a warm bath. Soak for ten minutes.

Blend six drops of lavender and six drops of eucalyptus into four ounces of carrier oil. Massage into temples, across the forehead, and into the back of the neck. Also try peppermint oil.

Mood Swings

Most useful: bergamot, clary sage, cypress, geranium, juniper, lavender, lemon, mandarin, orange (bitter), peppermint, rose, rosemary

Also try: coriander, rosewood

Recommended application: vaporizer, inhalation

Morning Sickness

Most useful: petitgrain, mandarin, sweet orange

Also try: melissa

Recommended application: vaporization, inhalation

Put a few drops of petitgrain and mandarin (or sweet orange) in a vaporizer or on a tissue to inhale when you feel symptoms. Put four drops of petitgrain, two drops of mandarin (or sweet orange), and one drop of sandalwood on a handkerchief and keep it on your pillow overnight. The aroma will linger until the morning, so the possibility of morning sickness will be lessened.

Muscle Cramps

Most useful: white birch, chamomile, lavender, rosemary

Also try: black pepper, coriander, ginger

Recommended application: massage

Nausea

Most useful: peppermint

Also try: black pepper, caraway, fennel, ginger, melissa, sandalwood, sweet orange, mandarin, petitgrain

Recommended application: bath, inhalation, vaporization, oil/lotion

Peppermint, caraway, and ginger are especially good for nausea associated with motion sickness. Mandarin and petitgrain are especially good for nausea associated with morning sickness (see **Morning Sickness.**)

Combine four drops of peppermint and four drops of ginger with a carrier oil. Massage this onto your chest to relieve nausea for motion sickness, or place a drop each of peppermint and ginger on a tissue or handkerchief. Inhale as needed.

Nervous System (to Balance)

Most useful: cypress, lavender, geranium, bergamot, rosemary

Also try: sage

Recommended application: massage, oil/lotion, bath

Create a massage oil using six drops of cypress and six drops of lavender in four ounces of carrier oil.

Put five drops of rosemary and five drops of sage in a warm bath. Soak ten minutes.

Palpitations

Most useful: ylang-ylang

Also try: bitter orange, sweet orange, orange blossom, rose

Recommended application: massage, inhalation

Perspiration

Most useful: cypress

Also try: citronella, lemongrass, petitgrain, pine, sage

Recommended application: oil/lotion, bath

Pimples

Most useful: lavender, tea tree, eucalyptus

Also try: bergamot

Recommended application: neat application

If you have sensitive skin, lavender is the least likely to cause skin irritation, but even still, use it sparingly. Before using any oil, especially on your face, it is wise to do a patch test.

Premenstrual Syndrome (PMS)

Most useful: bergamot, chamomile, clary sage, geranium, nutmeg, lavender, neroli, ylang-ylang, sweet marjoram, rose, tonka bean

Also try: carrot seed, orange blossom

Recommended application: massage, bath, vaporization

To a warm bath, add seven or eight drops of any of the oils mentioned on page 173. Soak for ten to fifteen minutes. Use any combination that works to relieve your premenstrual irritability. One suggestion is ylang-ylang with a drop or two of lavender.

Prickly Heat

Most useful: lavender, chamomile, eucalyptus

Also try: geranium

Recommended application: bath, compress

Psoriasis

Most useful: chamomile (German)

Also try: benzoin, bergamot, cajeput, lavender, niaouli

Recommended application: bath, oil/lotion

Add four or five drops to a warm bath to relieve the symptoms of psoriasis. After the bath, blend a ratio of one drop of chamomile to one ounce of your choice of carrier oil. Apply to the affected areas.

Mix $\frac{1}{2}$ ounce of grapeseed oil or sweet almond oil, fifteen drops of evening primrose oil, and five drops of German chamomile. Apply to the affected area.

Rashes

Most useful: chamomile, lavender

Also try: eucalyptus

Recommended application: bath, oil/lotion, compress

Respiratory Infection

Most useful: frankincense, lemon, niaouli, petitgrain, pine

Also try: rosewood, thyme

Recommended application: massage, vaporization, inhalation

Rheumatism

Most useful: white birch, chamomile, cypress, eucalyptus, juniper, lavender, marjoram, pine, rosemary

Also try: angelica, aniseed, basil, benzoin, cajeput, carrot seed, clove, coriander, fennel, lavandin, lemon, niaouli, nutmeg, black pepper, sage, thyme, vetivert, yarrow

Recommended application: massage, compress, bath

Scars

Most useful: lavender

Also try: cedarwood, frankincense, hyssop, myrrh, neroli, patchouli

Recommended application: oil/lotion

Scratches

Most useful: lavender

Also try: tea tree

Recommended application: oil/lotion, neat application (lavender, possibly tea tree)

Shingles

Most useful: eucalyptus, bergamot, geranium, peppermint, clove bud, sage, thyme

Also try: frankincense, niaouli

Recommended application: lotion/cream

Shock

Most useful: chamomile (Roman), lavender, melissa, neroli

Also try: lavandin, myrrh, petitgrain, ylang-ylang

Recommended application: massage, bath, vaporization

Sinusitis

Most useful: eucalyptus, peppermint, pine, tea tree

Also try: cajeput, cypress, geranium, ginger, niaouli, thyme, marjoram, hyssop, sage, rosemary

Recommended application: inhalation/steam, compress

Place one drop each of eucalyptus and geranium and two drops of rosemary on a handkerchief or tissue. Inhale the aroma.

Add ten drops of eucalyptus and ten drops of pine to a bowl of steaming water. Use the steam inhalation method. Another good combination is cypress and niaouli. Also try either of these combinations as a hot compress and apply to the sinus area.

Use a few drops of either peppermint, lavender, or eucalyptus in a cool-mist vaporizer overnight.

Smoking

Most useful: geranium, immortelle, lemon

Recommended application: inhalation, diffusion
Blend a three, two, one ratio of lemon, geranium, and immortelle. Blend and store in an amber bottle that you can keep with you. Inhale directly from the bottle or use a few drops in a diffuser when you crave that nicotine fix.

Sore Throat (Throat Infections)

Most useful: hyssop, cedarwood, eucalyptus, clary sage, sage, sandalwood, thyme

Also try: bergamot, cajeput, geranium, ginger, lavandin, lavender, myrrh, myrtle, niaouli, pine, tea tree, violet

Recommended application: vaporization, inhalation/steam, gargle, oil/lotion
Using a small amount of a carrier oil such as canola, safflower, or grapeseed, apply externally, covering the throat region. Then apply six or seven drops of sandalwood essential oil over the carrier oil and with gentle strokes, rub it into the skin.

Stress

Most useful: lavender, marjoram

Also try: grapefruit, cypress, geranium, petitgrain, fennel, neroli, melissa, chamomile, basil, bergamot, frankincense, hyssop, jasmine, lemon verbena, ylang-ylang, clary sage, rosemary

Recommended application: oil/lotion, bath, inhalation, diffusion

Either inhale the following mixture or use it as a massage oil for the upper body (face, neck, shoulders, chest, back): In one teaspoon of carrier oil, such as sweet almond oil, blend five drops of grapefruit, four drops of cypress, and two drops of geranium.

Place one drop of lavender and one drop of geranium on a tissue. Inhale this when you're feeling nervous. Also try substituting a drop of rosemary for the geranium.

Stretch Marks

Most useful: frankincense, geranium, myrrh, orange (bitter)

Also try: lavender, sweet orange, jasmine, neroli

Recommended application: oil/lotion

Stuffy Nose

Most useful: tea tree, rosemary

Recommended application: diffusion, inhalation

Sunburn

Most useful: lavender, chamomile

Also try: geranium, peppermint, eucalyptus, sandalwood

Recommended application: bath

Put twenty drops of chamomile and twenty drops of lavender into a cool bath. Soak ten minutes.

Add ten to twelve drops of lavender to four ounces of water in a spray bottle. Apply to your skin as needed.

Caution: If using peppermint oil, do not use more than one percent peppermint oil.

Sunstroke

Most useful: eucalyptus, lavender

Recommended application: bath

Throat Infections

See **Sore Throat.**

Tick Repellent

Most useful: peppermint

Also try: sweet marjoram

Recommended application: oil/lotion, spray

Mix five to ten drops of peppermint essential oil in one ounce of water in a spray bottle. Shake well. Spray around your ankles to help keep ticks at bay.

Tonsillitis

Most useful: thyme, lemon, niaouli, myrrh

Also try: bergamot, cedarwood, clary sage, clove, eucalyptus, geranium, hyssop, myrtle, rosemary, sage, tea tree

Recommended application: inhalation/steam, gargle

Try a gargle blend of ½ cup of warm water, ten drops of

tea tree oil, and ten drops of cedarwood oil. Use this four times a day.

Note: Serious conditions should be treated by a medical professional.

Urinary Tract Infection

Most useful: bergamot, chamomile, eucalyptus, benzoin, tea tree

Also try: sandalwood, juniper, thyme

Recommended application: bath, sitz bath, compress
Soak in a hot bath of eucalyptus and sandalwood (ten drops each) or juniper and thyme (ten drops each).

Vaginitis

Most useful: chamomile, clary, rose

Also try: bergamot, lavender, niaouli, tea tree, thyme

Recommended application: bath

Varicose Veins

Most useful: cypress, geranium

Also try: yarrow

Recommended application: oil/lotion
Combine ten drops of geranium and ten drops of cypress with four ounces of carrier oil. Massage gently around (not on) the veins, then apply oil very gently to the veins. It is recommended to stroke upward, toward the heart.

Vertigo

Most useful: lavender, peppermint

Also try: lavandin, melissa, violet

Recommended application: vaporization, inhalation/steam

Vomiting

Most useful: chamomile, lavender, peppermint, lemon, basil, black pepper, camphor, eucalyptus, frankincense, geranium, hyssop, juniper, marjoram, myrrh, patchouli, rosemary

Recommended application: inhalation, compresses, massage

Water Retention

Most useful: geranium, cypress, juniper

Recommended application: bath

Whooping Cough

Most useful: lavender, niaouli, tea tree

Also try: clary sage, hyssop, immortelle, rosemary, sage

Recommended application: massage, inhalation/steam

Wounds

Most useful: lavender, tea tree, myrrh

Also try: benzoin, bergamot, chamomile, eucalyptus, juniper, rosemary

Recommended application: neat application

All essential oils are antiseptic to some degree, but the ones mentioned above, especially lavender and tea tree, can be used directly on minor wounds. To avoid touching the wound, put a few drops of the essential oil on a sterile gauze pad and cover the wound. If a wound is very serious or needs stitches, however, seek appropriate medical treatment.

The therapeutic value of the essential oils listed in the preceding pages are a compilation of recommendations from many reference books, articles, and personal experiences of practicing aromatherapists.

Once again, these aromatherapy treatments are not meant as substitutes for seeking professional medical attention. It is also wise to consult a certified aromatherapist before using any essential oils for anything but simple home use.

PROPERTIES OF ESSENTIAL OILS

Here are some basic categories of essential oils. Note that there are many more oils that would fall into these groups, but those listed tend to be the most important and/or the most widely used for the particular effect.

Antidepressant oils: bergamot, benzoin, chamomile, clary sage, geranium, jasmine, lavender, melissa, neroli, petitgrain, orange, rose, sandalwood, ylang-ylang

Analgesic oils: bergamot, chamomile, lavender, marjoram, rosemary, aniseed, black pepper, cajeput, camphor, cinnamon, clove, coriander, eucalyptus, fennel, frankincense, geranium, ginger, juniper berry, niaouli, nutmeg, peppermint, tea tree

Anaphrodisiac oils: aniseed, marjoram, myrrh

Antiallergic oils: chamomile (German), hyssop, lavender

Antifungal oils: camphor, cinnamon, clove, eucalyptus, geranium, lavandin, myrrh, patchouli, tea tree, thyme, vetiver

Anti-infectious oils: bergamot, cajeput, camphor, chamomile, cinnamon, clary sage, clove, coriander, cypress, eucalyptus, geranium, hyssop, juniper, lavender, lemon, marjoram, neroli, niaouli, patchouli, peppermint, petitgrain, pine, rose, rosemary, rosewood, sage, tea tree, thyme, vetiver

Anti-inflammatory oils: benzoin, bergamot, calendula, chamomile (German), eucalyptus, geranium, immortelle, lavender, myrrh, peppermint, tea tree

Antiviral oils: basil, cajeput, camphor, cinnamon, clove, coriander, eucalyptus, hyssop, lavandin, lemon, niaouli, peppermint, rosewood, sage, tea tree, thyme

Aphrodisiac oils: rose, neroli (calming, soothing); clary sage, patchouli, ylang-ylang, jasmine, sandalwood, black pepper, cardamom (stimulating)

Astringent oils: cedarwood, cypress, frankincense, geranium, juniper, lemon, myrrh, patchouli, peppermint, rose, rosemary, rosewood, sandalwood

Bactericidal oils: aniseed, bergamot, cajeput, camphor, chamomile (Moroccan), cinnamon, clary sage, clove, coriander, cypress, eucalyptus, fennel, geranium, hyssop, lavandin, lemon, marjoram, neroli, niaouli, orange (sweet), petitgrain, rosemary, rosewood, sage, tea tree, thyme

Balancing oils: basil, cypress, frankincense, geranium, juniper, lavender, lemon, neroli, niaouli, orange (sweet), petitgrain, sage, sandalwood, ylang-ylang

Carminative oils: basil, bergamot, chamomile, caraway, cinnamon, fennel, ginger, lemon, marjoram, nutmeg, peppermint, rosemary

Cytophylactic (cell regenerating) oils: all essential oils to some extent, especially lavender, neroli, tea tree

Deodorizing oils: bergamot, clary sage, eucalyptus, lavender, neroli, juniper, cypress, ginger, nutmeg, thyme, sage, petitgrain, rosewood

Detoxifying oils: fennel, juniper, garlic, rose

Expectorant oils: basil, benzoin, bergamot, eucalyptus, fennel, marjoram, myrrh, tea tree, peppermint, niaouli, rosemary, sage, valerian, black pepper, frankincense, ginger, hyssop, juniper

Relaxant oils: basil, bergamot, cedarwood, chamomile, cinnamon, clary sage, cypress, frankincense, geranium, lavender, lemon, mandarin, marjoram, melissa, neroli, orange (sweet), petitgrain, sandalwood, valerian, ylang-ylang

Sedative oils: chamomile, lavender, bergamot, marjoram, neroli, benzoin, clary sage, rose, hyssop, jasmine, lemongrass, melissa, nutmeg, sandalwood, valerian

Stimulant oils: basil, black pepper, camphor, eucalyptus, rosemary, peppermint

Skin tonic oils: bergamot, camphor, cypress, geranium, juniper, peppermint, rose, rosemary

Uterine tonic oils: clary sage, jasmine, rose

Vulnerary (wound healing) oils: lavender, myrrh, tea tree, benzoin, bergamot, chamomile

CHAPTER 5

More Recipes

As any good chef will tell you, the art of cooking is inexact at best. When you ask for a recipe, you might hear, "Add a pinch of this, a dash of that." Aromatherapy recipes or blends are similar. Everyone has his or her own favorite blends, and the effects will be different for those who try them out. That's why custom blending in aromatherapy is so popular. One extra drop of this or that suited to your own preferences can make any blend more satisfying.

The following recipes are intended as guidelines. If you are a beginner to the world of essential oils, I recommend that you stick fairly closely to these recipes, as they are adapted from expert suggestions. In particular, some oils shouldn't be overused, and these recipes don't advocate using large amounts of potentially toxic oils. Once you feel more confident with how particular oils work together, however, and what makes you feel good, you should feel free to make your own blends. If in doubt, consult a professional aromatherapist.

INHALATIONS

Inhalation for Memory

Add equal parts rosemary and geranium to a diffuser.

Since inhaled aromas find their way to that part of the brain that controls memory and learning, the limbic system, this inhalation blend works particularly well. Geranium essential oil has antidepressant properties, and rosemary essential oil is a general mental stimulant. When you combine the two, they create a synergistic effect, where the combination is stronger than the individual components.

You can also inhale petitgrain essential oil directly from the bottle to enhance memory.

Sinus Inhalation Vaporizing Blend

½ oz. Professional Blend (see recipe on pages 52–53)
4 drops lavender
1 drop chamomile
3 drops rosemary
3 drops peppermint
4 drops eucalyptus

Courtesy of Elly Jesser-Yellin at Beyond the Crescent Moon, Great Neck, New York

For Anorexia

2 parts grapefruit
2 parts vanilla
1 part tonka bean

Use in an aroma lamp, bath oil, shower gel, skin lotion, or perfume to help regulate anorexia.

Adapted from information provided in *Complete Aromatherapy Handbook* by Suzanne Fischer-Rizzi, p. 202

For Anxiety

Mix together two, three, or four of these oils in equal parts: lavender, geranium, ylang-ylang, bergamot, and melissa. Use 10 to 12 drops in a diffuser or aroma lamp. Store mixture in an amber bottle for later use.

For Asthma

4 drops eucalyptus
2 drops lavender
2 drops myrrh
3 drops Roman chamomile

Use mixture in a diffuser or aroma lamp.

Caution: Since asthma sufferers usually have allergies, it is a good idea to be careful when using unfamiliar oils, especially for the first time.

For the Home or Office

For Clean, Fresh Air

Mix two drops of rosemary in a diffuser pot with a few drops of sweet orange.

Antiseptic Household Cleaner

15 drops peppermint
12 drops tea tree
20 drops lemon
8 drops lavender
½ oz. liquid castile soap

Fill 16-oz. spray bottle with water, add blend, and shake.

According to Sheryll Ryan, this blend also works as a room spray if you eliminate the castile soap. She notes that studies have shown that these oils will reduce the incidence of staph, strep, pneumococcus and other unpronounceable germs to almost zero.

Courtesy of Sheryll Ryan, District Director, National Association for Holistic Aromatherapy

For Cleaning and Brightening Musty Air

Fill a one oz. bottle with:

⅓ oz. geranium

⅓ oz. lavender

⅓ oz. lemon

Use blend as needed in a diffuser.

Marcy Freeman uses this blend in a diffuser in her office when she goes in after the weekend when the office building has been closed for a day. The other tenants in her building tell her they can't wait for her to come in on Mondays and start up her diffuser.

Courtesy of Marcy Freeman, Green Lotus Aromatherapy Company

Air Purification Formula

Clove	Rosemary
Cinnamon	Thyme
Lavender	6 oz. distilled water
Peppermint	1 oz. ethyl alcohol
Pine	

Mix three drops of each of the essential oils with the distilled water and ethyl alcohol. Place in a pump atomizer. Or blend five to ten drops of each of the oils and place in a vaporizer.

Formula excerpted from the aromatherapy certificate course offered by the Australasian College of Herbal Studies; courtesy of Dorene Peterson, Principal

Relaxation Blend

Add a few drops of any or all of the following oil(s) to an aroma lamp or diffuser or mix with water (three or four drops per cup of warm water) in a misting bottle and spray into the room:

Lavender
Mandarin
Cedarwood

Relaxation Blend #2

4 drops lemon
2 drops clary sage
1 drop vetiver

Add to a diffuser or aroma lamp.

Blend to Start Your Day on the Right Foot

3 drops rose
2 drops neroli

Add to an aroma lamp or diffuser.

To Lull You to Sleep

Add a few drops of any or all of the following oil(s) to an aroma lamp or diffuser or mix with water (three or four drops per cup of warm water) in a misting bottle and spray into the room.

Geranium
Mimosa
Roman chamomile
Rose
Neroli

To Soothe Stress

2 drops rose
4 drops lavender

Add to a diffuser or aroma lamp.

Stay Awake (but Calm) Blend

4 drops rosemary
2 drops sweet orange or mandarin

Add to diffuser or aroma lamp. (Better than caffeine!)

Sensual Blend

Add a few drops of any or all of the following oil(s) to an aroma lamp or diffuser or mix with water (three or four drops per cup of warm water) in a misting bottle and spray into the room.

Jasmine
Ylang-ylang
Sandalwood
Cinnamon
Patchouli

Creativity and Comfort Blend

2 drops iris
1 drop tonka bean
2 drops rose

Add to diffuser or aroma lamp.

(Note: Iris essential oil is quite rare and expensive. Its violet-like aroma, however, is believed to stir creative thoughts.)

Optimism Blend

2 drops neroli
8 drops grapefruit

Add to diffuser or aroma lamp.

Inhalation to Combat Fatigue and Keep Your Wits Sharp

Add a few drops of any or all of the following oil(s) to an aroma lamp or diffuser or mix with water (three or four drops per cup of warm water) in a misting bottle and spray into the room.

Lemon verbena
Peppermint
Juniper

Blend to Increase Concentration

6 drops hyssop
2 drops balm
1 drop mint
1 drop lime

Add to diffuser or aroma lamp.

SKIN AND HAIR CARE BLENDS

For the Face

Acne Formula

½ oz. sweet almond oil (carrier)
5 drops bergamot
2 drops juniper
2 drops lavender
1 drop peppermint
2 drops rose

Use in morning and evening.

Courtesy of Elly Jesser-Yellin at Beyond the Crescent Moon, Great Neck, New York

Nourishing Facial Balm
    5 drops geranium
    5 drops lavender
  3–5 drops frankincense
    ½ oz. unrefined or natural jojoba oil

Marcy Freeman likes this blend because it contains simple ingredients and you won't go broke making it.

Courtesy of Marcy Freeman, Green Lotus, Aromatherapy Company

For the Hair

Hair Loss Tonic Oil
   20 drops rosemary
   20 drops lavender
   10 drops basil

Mix the oils together in a ½-oz. amber or opaque bottle. Massage a few drops into your scalp nightly or apply a few drops to your hairbrush. According to Dorene Peterson of the Australasian College of Herbal Studies, this oil is wonderful for adding shine to your hair and stimulating growth. It does not leave your hair lank and greasy.

Formula excerpted from the aromatherapy certificate course offered by the Australasian College of Herbal Studies; courtesy of Dorene Peterson, Principal

For the Body

Dry, Scaly Skin Formula for Men*
    ½ oz. Professional Blend (see recipe on page 52–53)
    8 drops cedarwood
    6 drops chamomile
    4 drops lavender

1 drop patchouli
1 drop rose

Courtesy of Elly Jesser-Yellin at Beyond the Crescent Moon, Great Neck,
New York

Dry, Scaly Skin Formula for Women*

½ oz. Professional Blend (see recipe on page 52–53)
5 drops clary sage
2 drops jasmine
2 drops rosemary
2 drops rose
2 drops sandalwood

Courtesy of Elly Jesser-Yellin at Beyond the Crescent Moon, Great Neck,
New York

Body Oil for Dermatitis and Eczema

10 drops lavender
5 drops Roman chamomile
5 drops bergamot
5 drops neroli
2 oz. carrier oil, such as sweet almond oil

Apply to body after a warm bath.

Body Oil for Dry Skin

10 drops lavender
10 drops chamomile
10 drops neroli
10 drops rosemary
10 drops carrot seed
2 oz. carrier oil, such as sweet almond or sesame oil

Apply to damp skin after daily bath or shower.

*The women's formula contains more expensive oils, so the men's formula
can really be unisex.

For Dry, Brittle Nails

6 drops lavender
6 drops bay
6 drops sandalwood
6 oz. warm carrier oil (sesame or soy)

Combine ingredients. Soak for approximately 15 minutes. Treat one or two times per week.

BODY OILS/LOTIONS AND RUBS

Bronchitis Chest Rub Formula

½ oz. Professional Blend (see recipe on page 52–53)
5 drops eucalyptus
2 drops pine needle
2 drops hyssop (can be hazardous—ask a licensed aromatherapist about using hyssop)
1 drop lavender

Blend ingredients. Use as a chest rub.

Courtesy of Elly Jesser-Yellin at Beyond the Crescent Moon, Great Neck, New York

For Anxiety

Mix together two, three, or four of these oils in equal parts: lavender, geranium, ylang-ylang, bergamot, and melissa. Add six drops of this blend to a hot bath.

For Asthma

4 drops eucalyptus
3 drops Roman chamomile
2 drops myrrh
2 drops lavender
⅛ oz. olive oil

Blend ingredients. Use as a chest rub.

Caution: Since asthma sufferers usually have allergies, it is a good idea to be careful when using unfamiliar oils, especially for the first time.

Salve for Hemorrhoids

    2 drops lavender
    1 drop geranium
    1 ounce carrier oil

Blend mixture and use as a topical ointment after each bath or bowel movement.

Poor Circulation Oil

    8 drops juniper
   10 drops rosemary
    6 drops camphor
   50 ml (1.7 oz) carrier oil

Blend the essential oils with the base oil and apply externally as needed.

Formula excerpted from the aromatherapy certificate course offered by the Australasian College of Herbal Studies; courtesy of Dorene Peterson, Principal

Stretch Mark Oil (Kathy's Tummy Oil)

   15 drops jasmine
   25 drops sweet orange
   10 drops frankincense
   25 drops lavender
    5 drops galbanum*
    1 oz. cold-pressed virgin olive oil

*(Note: Galbanum essential oil, which is extracted by steam-distillation from a resinoid, can be used externally to treat a number of "women's" ailments. At one time, the plant was known as "mother's resin.")

This oil was developed by Marcia Elston of Samara Botane in Seattle for a friend's daughter when she had her first baby, and hence, to her dismay, her first stretch marks. This synergy concentrate should be applied moderately but often to help the skin recondition after pregnancy.

Courtesy of Marcia Elston, Samara Botane, Seattle, Washington

Muscle Ache Rub

   12 drops black pepper oil
    6 drops marjoram
    6 drops juniper
    6 drops ginger
    1 cup sweet almond oil

Combine the oils. Rub the blend into the affected area.

Formula excerpted from the aromatherapy certificate course offered by the Australasian College of Herbal Studies; courtesy of Dorene Peterson, Principal

Liniment Formula

   30 drops bay oil
   15 drops nutmeg oil
    9 drops black pepper oil
    1 cup peanut oil

Blend all oils together. Peanut oil can be replaced by another vegetable oil, such as sweet almond or grapeseed. However, peanut oil has a traditional reputation for its effectiveness to reduce the pain of arthritis and rheumatism.

Formula excerpted from the aromatherapy certificate course offered by the Australasian College of Herbal Studies; courtesy of Dorene Peterson, Principal

MASSAGE OILS

Massage Oil for Severe Backache
  3 drops chamomile
  3 drops ginger or black pepper
  3 drops white birch
  3 drops rosemary (eucalyptus can be substituted)
12 drops lavender
 ½ oz. carrier oil

Combine ingredients. Following a hot bath, massage the blend into the affected area. Use daily, as needed.

Minor Backache
Follow same recipe, but use only two drops of each essential oil. Mix in ½ ounce of carrier oil.

Following a hot bath, massage the blend into the affected area. Use daily, as needed.

Massage Oil for Muscle Aches
  6 drops lavender
  4 drops juniper
  2 drops rosemary
  4 oz. carrier oil, such as soy

Blend ingredients. Apply to sore muscles.

Massage Oil for Arthritis
  6 drops chamomile
  6 drops rosemary
  4 oz. carrier oil, such as sweet almond oil, avocado oil, or sesame oil

Combine ingredients. Rub into sore joints.

Massage Oil to Relieve Tension

6 drops lavender
4 drops chamomile
2 drops vetiver
4 oz. carrier oil, such as soy oil

Combine ingredients. Apply to body.

Massage Oil to Improve Circulation

6 drops lavender
4 drops rosemary
2 drops vetiver
4 oz. carrier oil, such as soy or sesame

Combine ingredients. Apply to body.

Massage Oil for Constipation

6 drops rosemary
6 drops thyme
1 oz. carrier oil, such as olive oil or almond oil

Combine ingredients. Gently massage abdominal area with the oil in a circular motion, starting with the right side.

High Blood Pressure Massage Oil

1 drop immortelle
2 drops chamomile
10 drops lavender
1 oz. carrier oil, such as sweet almond oil or sunflower

Combine ingredients. Massage into the area below the collarbone before you go to sleep.

Indigestion Massage Oil

4 drops peppermint
4 drops marjoram
4 drops coriander

4 drops fennel
4 drops basil
1 oz. olive or almond oil

Combine ingredients. Massage gently into the abdominal area.

Muscle Cramp Massage Oil
3 drops chamomile
3 drops white birch
3 drops rosemary
3 drops ginger
8 drops lavender
½ oz. sweet almond oil, grapeseed oil, or avocado oil

Combine ingredients. Massage into the muscles following a warm bath.

Seductive Massage Oil (Sheherazade's Seduction)
12–15 drops frankincense *(Boswellia carteri)*
4 drops ginger *(Zingiber officinale)*
3 drops coriander *(Coriandrum sativum)*
1 drop ylang-ylang extra *(Cananga odorata)*
2 oz. sweet almond oil

Combine ingredients.

Sheryll Ryan recalls that the first client who used this spicy, sensual blend was married to a workaholic surgeon. After using this blend in a massage for him, the doctor made it home early five nights in a row. The client now calls it her lucky blend.

Note: Botanical names referenced at the request of Sheryll Ryan.

Courtesy of Sheryll Ryan, District Director, National Association for Holistic Aromatherapy

Stress-Reducing Massage Formula

  6 drops anise
  6 drops rose
  6 drops nutmeg
  ½ cup sweet almond oil

Combine ingredients.

Formula excerpted from the aromatherapy certificate course offered by the Australasian College of Herbal Studies; courtesy of Dorene Peterson, Principal

Euphoria Massage Formula

  6 drops benzoin
  6 drops rose
  6 drops sandalwood
  ½ cup sweet almond oil

Combine ingredients.

Formula excerpted from the aromatherapy certificate course offered by the Australasian College of Herbal Studies; courtesy of Dorene Peterson, Principal

FOOT SOAKS

For Foot Odor

  10 drops lemon
   2 oz. water
Juice of 1 fresh lemon

Combine ingredients. Apply thoroughly to feet.

Soak for Foot Aches and Pain

  10 drops juniper
  10 drops lavender
   2 quarts warm water

Combine ingredients. Soak feet for ten minutes.

Soak for Foot Pain Due to Gout

   10 drops juniper
   10 drops rosemary
    2 quarts cold water

Combine ingredients. Soak feet for ten minutes.

AROMATIC BATH RECIPES

Don't forget to always mix the oils first with vegetable oil, honey, vodka, whole milk, or cream. Oils should be added after you've been in the bath long enough to adjust to the temperature.

Bath Oil Blend

    4 oz. Professional Blend (see pages 52–53)
   12 drops chamomile
    6 drops lavender
    6 drops sweet orange or mandarin

According to aromatherapist Elly Jesser-Yellin of Beyond the Crescent Moon, this blend is great for relaxation. It's excellent for the skin and just makes you feel really good. It can also be used as a body oil after the bath. Keep this blend on hand.

Courtesy of Elly Jesser-Yellin at Beyond the Crescent Moon, Great Neck, New York

Migraine Headache Bath #1

    7 drops lavender
    7 drops eucalyptus

Add to a warm bath. Mix well. Soak for ten minutes.

Migraine Headache Bath #2
    8 drops chamomile
    7 drops rosemary

Add to a warm bath. Mix well. Soak for ten minutes.

Stimulating Morning Bath #1
    4 drops rosemary
    2 drops petitgrain

Add to a warm bath. Mix well. Soak for ten minutes.

Stimulating Morning Bath #2
    3 drops rosemary
    3 drops bergamot

Add to a warm bath. Mix well. Soak for ten minutes.

Cleansing/Refreshing Bath #1
    3 drops lemon
    3 drops geranium
Juice of 1 fresh lemon (optional)

Add to a warm bath. Mix well. Soak for ten minutes.

Cleansing/Refreshing Bath #2
    3 drops thyme
    2 drops rosemary
    1 drop lavender
    1 drop peppermint

Add to a warm bath. Mix well. Soak for ten minutes.

Comforting and Reviving Bath
    4 drops lavender
    3 drops peppermint

Add to a warm bath. Mix well. Soak for ten minutes.

Muscle Relaxing Bath #1

4 drops rosemary
2 drops marjoram
3 drops lavender

Add to a warm bath. Mix well. Soak for ten minutes.

Muscle Relaxing Bath #2

4 drops rosemary
2 drops marjoram
3 drops Roman chamomile

Add to a warm bath. Mix well. Soak for ten minutes.

Cheering Bath

7 drops geranium
5 drops bergamot
2 drops lavender

Add to a warm bath. Mix well. Soak for about ten minutes.

Morning Bath for Colds and Flu

3 drops lavender
2 drops rosemary
2 drops thyme

Add to a warm bath. Mix well. Soak for ten minutes.

Bath for Colds and Flu

4 drops rosemary
2 drops verbena

Add to a warm bath. Mix well. Soak for ten minutes.

Bath for Common Cold

   3 drops lemon oil
   1 drop eucalyptus
   2 drops thyme
   2 drops tea tree

Add to a hot bath. Mix well. Soak for ten minutes. Deeply inhale the aroma.

Bath for Common Cold, Flu, or Bronchitis #1

   7 drops pine
   7 drops eucalyptus

Add to a hot bath. Mix well. Soak for ten minutes. Deeply inhale the aroma.

Bath for Common Cold, Flu, or Bronchitis #2

   7 drops sandalwood
   6 drops camphor

Add to a hot bath. Mix well. Soak for ten minutes. Deeply inhale the aroma.

Bath for Depression or Fear #1

   4 drops clary sage
   2 drops bergamot
   6 drops melissa
   4 drops basil

Add to a warm bath. Mix well. Soak for ten minutes.

Bath for Depression #2

   7 drops neroli
   7 drops basil

Add to a warm bath. Mix well. Soak for ten minutes.

Bath for Depression #3

   7 drops marjoram
   7 drops ylang-ylang

Add to a warm bath. Mix well. Soak for ten minutes.

After-Work Relaxing Bath

   2 drops lavender
   1 drop geranium
   1 drop neroli

Add to a warm bath. Mix well. Soak for ten minutes.

Sitz Bath for Hemorrhoids #1

   8 drops lavender
   7 drops juniper

Add to a shallow, hot bath. Mix well. Soak for ten minutes.

Sitz Bath for Hemorrhoids #2

   6 drops cypress
   6 drops chamomile

Add to a shallow, hot bath. Mix well. Soak for ten minutes.

Bath for Nervousness or Overexcitement

   3 drops geranium
   2 drops basil
   2 drops lavender
   2 drops clary sage
   3 drops orange
   1 drop jasmine

Add to a warm bath. Mix well. Soak for ten minutes.

Relaxation Bath

   3 drops lavender
   2 drops clary sage
   2 drops mandarin

Add to a warm bath. Mix well. Soak for ten minutes.

Soothing Bath

   4 drops lavender
   6 drops tangerine
   2 drops marjoram

Add to a warm bath. Mix well. Soak for ten minutes.

Tension-Reliever Bath

  10 drops vetiver
  10 drops lavender

Add to a warm bath. Mix well. Soak for ten minutes.

Relaxing Bath

   2 drops clary sage
   2 drops ylang-ylang

Add to the bath after it is full; mix the oils well and immerse yourself for a wonderful, relaxing soak.

Formula excerpted from the aromatherapy certificate course offered by the Australasian College of Herbal Studies; courtesy of Dorene Peterson, Principal

Bath for Mental Confusion #1

   6 drops melissa
   4 drops bergamot
   6 drops lemon
   2 drops lemongrass
   2 drops lavender

Add to a warm bath. Mix well. Soak for ten minutes.

Bath for Mental Confusion #2

    4 drops rosewood
    4 drops patchouli

Add to a warm bath. Mix well. Soak for ten minutes.

Bath for Shock #1

    4 drops clary sage
    2 drops marjoram
    2 drops rose
    2 drops ylang-ylang

Add to a warm bath. Mix well. Soak for ten minutes.

Bath for Shock #2

    4 drops cypress
    2 drops cedarwood
    2 drops sandalwood

Add to a warm bath. Mix well. Soak for ten minutes.

Bath for Kidneys/Urinary Infections

    10 drops eucalyptus
    10 drops sandalwood

Add to a hot bath. Mix well. Soak for ten minutes.

Extra-Relaxing Bath

    10 drops lavender
    5 drops marjoram

Add to a warm bath. Mix well. Soak for about twenty minutes.

Marjoram is a sedative, so don't use more than five drops. You might fall asleep.

Caution: Marjoram should not be used when you are pregnant.

Self-Confidence Bath
   4 drops ylang-ylang
   4 drops marjoram
   3 drops jasmine

Add to a warm bath. Mix well. Soak for ten minutes.

Colds and Flu Bath
   5 drops eucalyptus
   5 drops peppermint
   4 drops lavender
   7 drops thyme (optional—use if your chest is congested)

Add to a warm bath. Mix well. Soak for ten minutes.

Cool Sunburn Bath
   10 drops chamomile
   10 drops lavender

Add to a cool bath. Mix well. Soak for ten minutes.

Water Retention Bath
   6 drops geranium
   6 drops juniper
   6 drops cypress

Add to a warm bath. Mix well. Soak for about ten minutes.

References

Ackerman, Diane, *A Natural History of the Senses,* Vintage Books (1990).

Blake-Weisenthal, D., "What the Nose Knows," *Vegetarian Times,* Oct. 1992, 95.

Brody, Jane E., "Elderly and Can't Sleep? Try Scent of Lavender," *New York Times,* Sept. 13, 1995, C9.

Castleman, Michael, *Nature's Cures,* Rodale Press, Inc. (1996).

Clayton, Craig, and Virginia McCullough, *A Consumer's Guide to Alternative Health Care,* Adams Publishing (1995).

Cunningham, Scott, *Magical Aromatherapy,* Llewellyn Publications, Inc. (1989).

Davis, Patricia, *Aromatherapy: An A–Z,* C. W. Daniel (1988).

Dodt, Colleen K., *The Essential Oils Book: Creating Personal Blends for Mind & Body,* Storey Communications, Inc. (1996).

Fettner, Ann Tucker, *Potpourri, Incense and Other Fragrant Concoctions,* Workman Publishing Company (1977).

Fischer-Rizzi, Suzanne, *Complete Aromatherapy Handbook: Essential Oils for Radiant Health,* Sterling Publishing Company (1990).

Gattefosse, René-Maurice, *Gattefosse's Aromatherapy,* C. W. Daniel Co., Ltd. (1937).

Gottlieb, Bill, ed., *New Choices in Natural Healing,* Rodale Press (1995).

Griffin, K., "A Whiff of Things to Come," *Health,* Nov./Dec. 1992, 34.

Jackson, Judith, *Scentual Touch: A Personal Guide to Aromatherapy,* Henry Holt and Company (1986).

Keller, Erich, *Aromatherapy Handbook for Beauty, Hair, & Skin Care,* Healing Arts Press (1991).

Lavabre, Marcel, *The Aromatherapy Workbook,* Healing Arts Press (1990).

Lawless, Julia, *The Illustrated Encyclopedia of Essential Oils: The Complete Guide to the Use of Oils in Aromatherapy and Herbalism,* Element Books (1995).

Morris, Edwin T., *Fragrance: The Story of Perfume from Cleopatra to Chanel,* Charles Scribner's Sons (1984).

Murray Willeford, Lynn, "Home Sacred Home: Fill a Room with Healing Scents," *New Age Journal,* Jan./Feb. 1996, 65–69.

Muryn, Mary, "Water Magic," *New Age Journal,* Jan./Feb. 1996, 99–102.

Price, Shirley, *The Aromatherapy Workbook: Understanding Essential Oils from Plant to Bottle,* Thorson's, an imprint of Harper Collins Publishers (1993).

Rose, Jeanne, *The Aromatherapy Book,* North Atlantic Press (1992).

Tisserand, Maggie, *Aromatherapy for Women: A Practical Guide to Essential Oils for Health and Beauty,* Healing Arts Press (1988).

Tisserand, Robert B., *The Art of Aromatherapy: The Healing and Beautifying Properties of the Essential Oils of Flowers and Herbs,* Healing Arts Press (1977).

Valnet, Jean, *The Practice of Aromatherapy.* C. W. Daniel Co. (1982).

Worwood, Valerie Ann. *The Complete Book of Essential Oils & Aromatherapy,* New World Library (1991).

Resources

American Aromatherapy Association
PO Box 1222
Fair Oaks, CA 95628
(916) 965-7546

American Association of Naturopathic Physicians
PO Box 2579
Kirkland, WA 98083-2579
(206) 827-6035

American Foundation for Alternative Health Care, Research and Development
25 Landfield Avenue
Monticello, NY 12701
(914) 794-8181

American Holistic Medical Association
2727 Fairview Avenue East, Suite B
Seattle, WA 98102
(206) 322-6842

American Massage Therapy Association
National Information Office
1130 West North Shore Avenue
Chicago, IL 60626
(312) 761-2682

Aromatherapy Organisations Council
3 Latymer Close
Braybrook
Market Harbourough
Leicester LE16 8LN
U.K.
*This is an umbrella organi-
zation that represents
fourteen associations and
societies dealing with
aromatherapy.*

Aromatherapy Quarterly
PO Box 421
Iverness, CA 94937-0421
(415) 663-9519
Fax: (415) 663-9128

Aromatherapy Seminars
1830 S. Robertson
Boulevard, #203
Los Angeles, CA 90035
(800) 677-2368

The Aromatic Thymes
75 Lakeview Parkway
Barrington, IL 60010
Fax: (847) 526-8432

The Australasian College of Herbal Studies
PO Box 57
Lake Oswego, OR 97034
(800) 48-STUDY

International Federation of Aromatherapists
Stamford House
2-4 Chiswick High Road
London, England W4 1TH
0181-742 2605
Subscription available for
The Aromatherapy Times

The International Journal of Aromatherapy
Robert Tisserand
PO Box 746
Hove, East Sussex
England BN3 3XA
01273 772479
Fax: 01273 329811

International Society of Professional Aromatherapists
Hinckley and District
Hospital and Health Care
The Annex
Mount Road
Hinckley, Leicestershire
LE10 1AG, England
0455 637987
Fax: 0455 890956

National Association for Holistic Aromatherapy
PO Box 17622
Boulder, CO 80308-7622
(800) 566-6735

**Pacific Institute of
Aromatherapy**
PO Box 606
San Raphael, CA 94915
(415) 459-3998

**Jeanne Rose
Aromatherapy**
219 Carl Street
San Francisco, CA 94117
(415) 564-6337

**The New England Center
for Aromatherapy**
60 Myrtle Street, Suite 1
Boston, MA 02114
(617) 720-4585

**Smell and Taste
Treatment and
Research Foundation**
Water Tower Place
845 North Michigan
Avenue, Suite 990W
Chicago, IL 60611
(312) 938-1047
*Headed by Alan Hirsch,
M.D., the facility
conducts experiments
related to disorders of
smell and taste.*

ESSENTIAL OIL SOURCES

The following sources are generally regarded as dealing in
high-quality oils, as well as distributing various aromatherapy-
related products and blends.

Aroma Vera Inc.
5901 Rodeo Drive
Los Angeles, CA 90016-
4312
(800) 669-9514 or (310)
280-0407

Aromaland
RR 20, Box 29 AL
Santa Fe, NM 87501
(800) 933-5267

Aura Cacia
PO Box 399
Weaverville, CA 96093
(800) 437-3301

**The Essential Oil
Company**
PO Box 206
Lake Oswego, OR 97034
(800) 729-5912

Fleur Aromatherapy
Pembroke Studios
Pembroke Road
Muswell Hill
London, England N10 2JE
081-444-7424 081

Frontier Co-Op Herbs
3021 78th St.
PO Box 299
Norway, IA 52318
(800) 669-3275

**Jeanne Rose
  Aromatherapy**
219 Carl Street
San Francisco, CA 94117

Lavender Lane
5321 Elkhorn Boulevard
Sacramento, CA 95842

**Liberty Natural Products,
  Inc.**
8120 SE Stark Street
Portland, OR 97215

(800) 289-8427 or
  (503) 256-1227
Fax: (503) 256-1182
E-mail:
  liberty@teleport.com
Web:
  http://www.teleport.com/
  ~liberty

Original Swiss Aromatics
28 Paul Street, Suite F
PO Box 6842
San Rafael, CA 94903
(415) 459-3998

**Shirley Price
  Aromatherapy Ltd.**
Essentia House
Upper Bond Street
Hinckley, Leicestershire
England LE10 1RS
01455 615466
Fax: 01455 615054

OTHER AROMATIC PRODUCTS

Origins
767 Fifth Avenue
New York, NY
(800) ORIGINS or
  (800) 723-7310 (to order)

Aveda Corporation
400 Central Avenue
  Southeast
Minneapolis, MN 55414
(800) 448-6265

INTERNET SITES

Mailing Lists
listserv@idma.com

Newsgroups
alt.aromatherapy
alt.folklore.aromatherapy

Web Sites

There are currently almost 400 entries on the World Wide Web that deal with aromatherapy. Here are just a few from professional organizations, wholesalers, retailers, and distributors, along with the description as listed on the Internet.

http://www.eskimo.com/~hhnews/naha (National Association for Holistic Aromatherapy)
http://www.eskimo.com/~joanne (Bassett Aromatherapy WWW Catalog)
http://www.htp.com/glac/welcome.html (Green Lotus Aromatherapy Company)
http:/www.teleport.com/~synergy/indexl.html (Aroma Therapy/A Synergy of Healing)
http:www.aromavera.com (Aromatherapy Products)
http://www.halcyon.com/kway (Ancient Healing Art—Scentsible Aromatherapy)
http://www.demon.co.uk/murderon/fragrant (The Guide to Aromatherapy)
http://www.pitt.edu/~cbw/altm.html (Alternative Medicine Homepage)

http://www.teleport.com/~liberty (Liberty National Products, Inc.)
http://www.wingedseed.com/samara (Samara Botane, Seattle, WA)

To search for aromatherapy-related Web sites, try using key search words: *aromatherapy, alternative medicine, essential oils, herbs.*

About the Author

Robyn M. Feller, a writer and editor, is the author of *Everything You Need to Know about Peer Pressure* and *The Complete Bartender.* She lives with her husband, Paul Sundick, in Great Neck, New York.

eczema
Psoriasis
dermatitis
Inflamed skin
Skin irritations
rash
hair
Chamomile
Cedar
scalp
dandruff
eczema